Alternative Medicine - New Insights

Edited by Cengiz Mordeniz

Published in London, United Kingdom

Alternative Medicine - New Insights
http://dx.doi.org/10.5772/intechopen.1003494
Edited by Cengiz Mordeniz

Contributors
Awal Prasetyo, Chadi Khatib, Daisy Jepkosgei Kipkemoi, Durga Prasad Beda, Erika Loučanová, Francis Omujal, Hendro Prabowo, Joseph Mukisa, Leonidas A. Johnson, Martina Nosáľová, Milind Nisargandha, Shweta Parwe, Veeresh Pratap

First published in London, United Kingdom, 2025 by IntechOpen
IntechOpen is the global imprint of INTECHOPEN LIMITED, registered in England and Wales, registration number: 11086078, 167-169 Great Portland Street, London, W1W 5PF, United Kingdom

For EU product safety concerns: IN TECH d.o.o., Prolaz Marije Krucifikse Kozulić 3, 51000 Rijeka, Croatia, info@intechopen.com or visit our website at intechopen.com.

British Library Cataloguing-in-Publication Data
A catalogue record for this book is available from the British Library

Alternative Medicine - New Insights
Edited by Cengiz Mordeniz
p. cm.
Print ISBN 978-0-85014-802-2
Online ISBN 978-0-85014-801-5
eBook (PDF) ISBN 978-0-85014-803-9

If disposing of this product, please recycle the paper responsibly.

Meet the editor

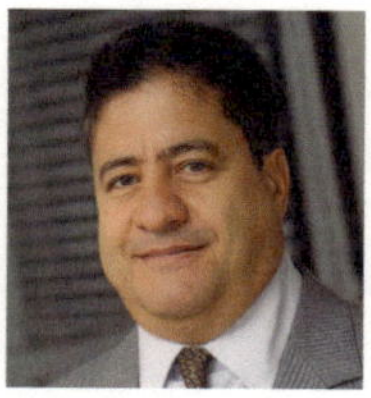

Professor Dr. Cengiz Mordeniz is a member of the Medical Faculty in the Department of Anesthesiology and Intensive Care and Pain Medicine, at the Tekirdag Namik Kemal University in Turkey. He also works at the Traditional and Complementary Medicine Center of the University Hospital, performing acupuncture, digital homeopathy, hirudotherapy, cupping therapy, apitherapy and acupuncture, and ozone therapy. He is interested in vibrational and informational medicine to predict pathologies in energetic biofields in advance and modulate them through frequency therapies.

Contents

Preface

Human beings are biological, psychological, social, and spiritual beings. However, modern medicine considers the person just as a somatic being and treats them only when they have certain symptoms. The person presenting the symptoms has to be taken as a particular case, and the symptoms' root cause must be detected. But what happens is that they usually receive a pharmacological receipt to overcome the symptoms transiently. Every speciality approaches from their part of the body. The root cause is often missed, and the person is tagged with many standardized diseases and receives medicine for each symptom. If there is a side effect, new medicine is added. Typically, these medications require long-term, sometimes lifelong management. If a drug proves ineffective, it's combined with higher doses or replaced with a different one. The same approach is applied to manage side effects.

So, there is a need to approach the problem holistically. All the symptoms must be considered simultaneously to detect the leading cause using psychological, social, and spiritual approaches. Epigenetically, it is found that everyone has particular metabolic cycles, which should be considered for every person. Personalized medicine aims at everyone personally. There is no disease but only the patient. Current management treats everyone as a patient, categorizing them with one or more diseases. The individual is no longer seen as a unique person but as a standardized digital identity, simply given drugs to relieve symptoms.

To cure the disease, a person must be advised about every lifestyle aspect. The future of medicine will focus on lifestyle changes that encourage proactive health rather than waiting for symptoms to appear. It's now understood that by the time symptoms show up, the disease may have already begun, sometimes even years earlier—such as in Alzheimer's, where it can start up to 10 years before symptoms emerge. The reason is that biochemical and microbiological methods and imaging technology are used in the algorithmic approach. Those methods detect some biomarkers or images. When the biomarkers or the image are detectable, it means that the disease is advanced. New techniques, such as energy-based and vibrational medicine, are emerging as innovative approaches to healing. The goal is to detect diseases early and treat them at an energetic level without relying on drugs.

In the book, traditional methods are scientifically evaluated to integrate them with modern medicine, ensuring they are not just viewed as alternative treatments.

The first chapter overviews alternative medicine historically through science and religion and the concept of health and wellness, bringing up the lifestyle as the main core of health. The second chapter exposes innovations that are scientifically considered alternative methods.

The second section is reserved for the importance of nature and analyzes how nature affects health. The first chapter of the section recalls the natural way of staying healthy.

Living naturally will appear as lifestyle medicine. Everybody should regulate their lifestyle with a natural diet, regular exercise and stress coping. For example, living or passing time in nature or a forest helps to be healthy. The second chapter of the second section also emphasizes some rituals in a green environment and the effect of nature on lifestyles related to health and wellness.

Most drugs are derived from plants and are used to manage disease and prevent the symptoms before they manifest. The plant itself, its odour, or its vapour can all be used in different forms of treatment. When the plant is used directly, it's called phytotherapy. If its aroma is utilized, it's known as aromatherapy. When minimal doses are used, it's referred to as homeopathy. If specific flowers are used, they are called Bach flowers. If certain combinations of minerals are used, they are known as Schüssler salts, among other remedies.

In the third section, aromatherapy is reviewed through history and the therapeutic application of phytochemicals in the first chapter. The second chapter of the section takes as an example the management of Alzheimer's disease with plants and new insights into alternative medicine.

The first chapter of the final section introduces and explains a new method using a graphite plate. The last chapter of this section and the book presents an example from one of the major traditional medicines, primarily Ayurveda from India, with a specific example for treating constipation.

As a result, the approach shifts from the allopathic method of merely suppressing symptoms to an epigenetic test that addresses biological, psychological, social, and spiritual factors, aiming for a personalized and holistic approach to medicine. In disease management, the focus should be on identifying the root cause, with consideration given to the energetic level. Energetic or vibrational medicine can potentially transform alternative treatments into integrative medicine grounded in scientific evidence.

Cengiz Mordeniz
Tekirdag Namik Kemal University,
Tekirdag, Turkey

Section 1

New Frontiers in Alternative Medicine

Chapter 1

A Particular Visual Enlightenment: A Refraction of Science, Religion, and Health on Wellness and Fullness of Life

Leonidas A. Johnson

Abstract

Western allopathic medicine, Traditional East Asian Medicine (TEAM), and Energy Medicine often use vastly different scientific-based methodologies, logic, and religious/spiritual paths in the pursuit of health, wellness, and ultimately, the fullness of life. Excellent physical health alone does not equate to an excellent quality of life. Healers who labor to put people in a position to grab all the gusto life has to offer should possess a tool that increases their ability to align, converge, and bring into focus scientific, religious/spiritual, and multiple medical health vantage points to promote wellness and the fullness of life outcome. *A Particular Visual Enlightenment (APVE)* is a metaphysical refraction, an optical tool, that aligns and converges the disciplines of science, religion/spirituality, and health with a focus on wellness and the fullness of life.

Keywords: phenomenal vision (PVis), mental vision, spiritual vision, spiritual health, metaphysical refraction, three dimensions of human existence (TDoHE), traditional east Asian medicine (TEAM), acupuncture, Yin and Yang theory, five-phase correspondence theory, salutogenic

1. Introduction

Refraction is a test included in a comprehensive eye exam to determine the best prescription to achieve the best visual acuity (BVA) for clear, comfortable, efficient, binocular vision. Physical vision involves central vision plus other things like peripheral vision, night vision, color vision, depth perception, contrast sensitivity, and low/high order aberration sensitivity.

Refraction is also defined as the bending of light. For learning purposes, refraction can also be defined as the art and science of using alignment and convergence to bring things into clear focus and improve vision, physical and metaphysical. A salutogenic perspective magnifies the idea of a wellness continuum ([1, 2], p. 44). Refraction of physical and metaphysical realities with a salutogenic depth of focus (DOF) on health and wellness using fullness of life (FOL) as a focal point would be a valuable

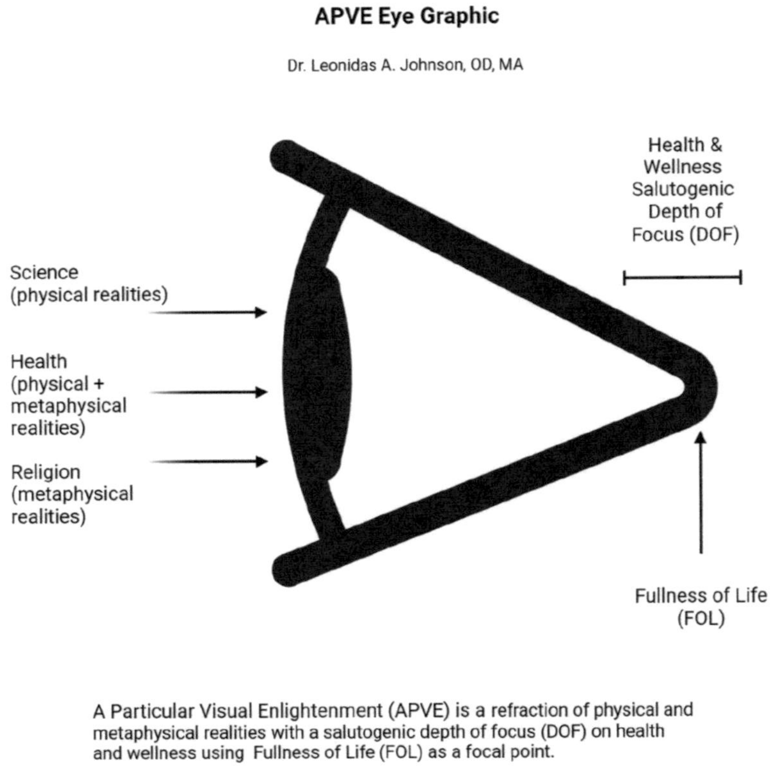

Figure 1.
APVE eye graphic.

individual and collective tool, particularly to healers (see **Figure 1**, i.e., APVE Eye Graphic illustration).

A Particular Visual Enlightenment (APVE) is a refraction of physical and metaphysical realities, a corrective lens-type tool in the form of a diagram that aligns and converges the disciplines of science, religion/spirituality, and health with a focus on the wellness continuum and fullness of life (see **Figure 2**, i.e., APVE FOL diagram). The refraction of physical and metaphysical realities, which incorporate the concepts of *Phenomenal Vision (PVis)* (i.e., the physical, mental, and spiritual phenomena of enlightenment), Three Dimensions of Human Existence (TDoHE) (i.e., body, soul, spirit), Traditional East Asian Medicine (TEAM) (i.e., Acupuncture, Herbal prescriptions, Tui Na Massage, Qigong), Yin-Yang Theory (YY-Theory), Five-phase Theory (FP-Theory), Universal Cause-Effect Paradigm (UCEP), with a focus on wellness and fullness of life, all in alignment with the Ancient of Days (AOD) (i.e., that which existed before time) and eternity, is collectively referred to as *A Particular Visual Enlightenment (APVE)*.

A Particular Visual Enlightenment (APVE), due to its unique structure and composition, can be likened to the flexibility and strength of a bamboo plant. The alignment and convergence of seemingly divergent and contradictory concepts in *A Particular Visual Alignment* require the mental flexibility of a gymnast and the convictional strength of an African bush elephant. Like a tender bamboo plant rooted in dry ground, *A Particular Visual Enlightenment (APVE)* is flexible and strong due to its unique structure and inspirational composition.

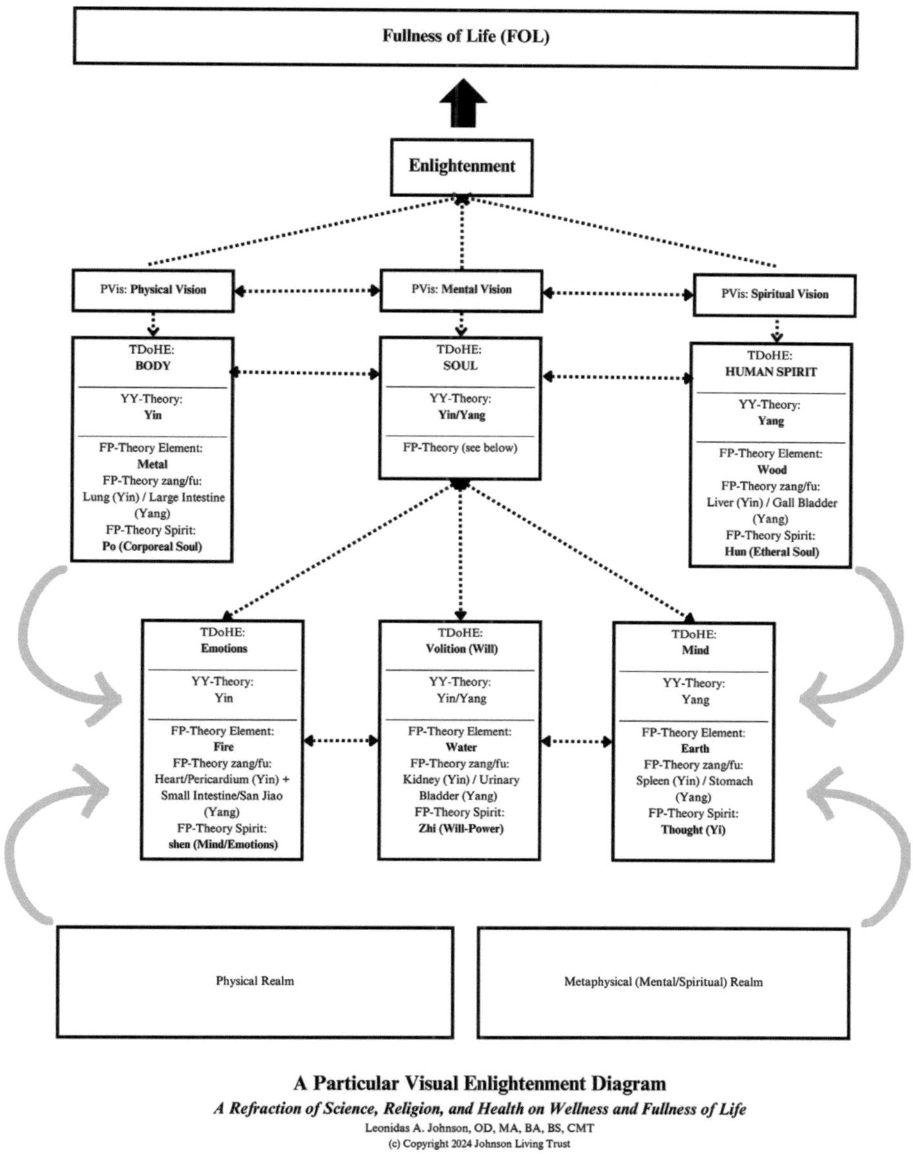

Figure 2.
APVE FOL diagram.

2. Discourse in metaphysical optics

2.1 The refraction of physical and metaphysical realities

The refraction of physical and metaphysical realities can be related to the art and science of optometric vision care. Physical realities relate to scientific methodology and metaphysical realities relate to the first causes of things and things that do not change, the origin of things and things that are eternal. The philosophical science of metaphysics includes the domains of psychology and religion/spirituality. Switching back-and-forth from physical to metaphysical realities and from realities that are physically visible to those that are physically invisible can easily be accomplished with comparison learning. Comparison is a powerful learning process that has been leveraged to improve learning in a variety of domains [3]. This exercise in comparison learning will help healers stretch toward the mark and high calling to do no harm in the pursuit of better health outcomes, improved wellness, and fullness of life (FOL).

It would be prudent to enter this refractive experience with a perusal of the art and science of bending of light and basic optics. A basic understanding of optics and the nature of light can, by comparative learning, lead to an understanding of physiological optics. An understanding of physiological optics can, by comparison learning, lead to an understanding of refractive and medical eye conditions. An understanding of physical refractive and medical eye conditions can, by comparison learning, lead to an understanding of metaphysical refractive and metaphysical medical eye conditions. An understanding of physical vision can, by comparison learning, lead to an understanding of mental vision. An understanding of mental vision can, by comparison learning, lead to an understanding of spiritual vision. A review of the physical refraction eye test can, by comparison learning, lead to an understanding of this refraction of physical and metaphysical realities. Why go through the iterations of comparison learning? This process reflects the art and science of using alignment and convergence to bring things into clear focus and improve vision.

Vision, what is it? Why focus on vision? Vision is key to unlocking the many mysteries of life. Vision is our most dominant physical sense.

> *Studies estimate that between 50 and 80 percent of the human brain is dedicated to various forms of visual processing, such as vision, visual memory, colors, shapes, movement, patterns, spatial awareness, and image recollection ([4], pp. xix, 14).*

The eye is an extension of the brain, and the brain is most efficient at processing physical information visually (i.e., in a visual format). Eye care specialists have learned that 80–85% of adult perception, learning, cognition, and activities in the physical world involve visual processing compared to 11% from hearing, 3.5% from smell, 1.5% from touch, and 1% from taste [5]. It is of no surprise that, via comparison learning, the brain can efficiently process information about nonphysical metaphysical realities in a visual format. *Vision transcends the domain of physical realities and serves as a conduit to the domain of metaphysical realities.*

2.2 Phenomenal vision (PVis)

Vision is three-dimensional and time is one-dimensional. Physical vision concerns how we see the physical world (outward look) and its reach in the temporal domain of past, present, and future is confined to the present. Mental vision concerns how we see ourselves (inward look) and its reach in the space–time continuum (past, present, future) is unrestricted. Spiritual vision concerns how we see ourselves in relationship to the world/universe (worldview) and transcends the space–time continuum with a reach from eternity to eternity.

The term *Phenomenal Vision (PVis)* emphasizes the importance vision plays in seeing physical and nonphysical metaphysical realities. *Phenomenal Vision (PVis)* is defined as *the physical, mental, and spiritual phenomena of enlightenment. Phenomenal Vision (PVis)* refers to the life-changing ability to take a general understanding of physical vision and compare that understanding to mental and spiritual vision ([6], p. 6). Application of phenomenal vision, vision that encompasses the physical, mental, and spiritual aspects of vision, can bring clarity to life, the fullness of life, and unlock mysteries of life ([6], pp. 5, 6). *Phenomenal vision (PVis)* gives us the ability to look from the various vantage points of science, religion/spirituality, and health traditions/disciplines to improve our decision-making strategy to better individual and collective health outcomes, improve wellness as defined by quality of life, and enter a state where we have access to all the gusto life has to offer, the fullness of life!

2.2.1 Mental vision

Light is electromagnetic radiation with a peculiar and paradoxical nature. Light behaves as a wave and as a particle. Light particles are photons without mass that move at the speed of light and have energy proportional to their frequency. Light waves typically travel in straight lines but when traveling from one medium like water to another medium like air, the speed of light changes causing light waves to bend, refract, at the interface between the two mediums. This phenomenon of refraction can be used to design highly complex optical systems or simple curved surfaces, like a convex lens, to cause the light waves to align and converge to a single focal point. A convex lens bends light waves toward the optical axis to a focal point located behind the lens. A concave lens bends light waves away from the optical axis to a virtual focal point located in front of the lens. An optical illusion can occur when light bends in a manner that deceives the eye, like a mirage of a desert oasis.

Principals of physical optics can be applied to the human eye. The eye is an optical system composed of living tissue that can align and converge light rays to a focal point on the retina. When principles of physical optics are applied to the eye, they are referred to as physiological optics vis comparison learning. If the focal point of an image is formed on the retina, there is no refractive error. If the focal point of an image is formed anterior to the retina, the refractive error is called myopia. Corrective minus powered lenses can be prescribed to move the focal point more posterior so that the image focuses on the retina. If an image is formed posterior to the retina, the refractive error is called hypermetropia. Corrective plus powered lenses can be prescribed to move the focal point more anterior so that the image focuses on the retina. If the eye curvature has a dual nature (two different curves 90 degrees apart instead of one single curvature), the image spreads between different focal points and the refractive error is called astigmatism. Corrective lenses that are bitoric in design can be prescribed to align and converge the two spread-out focal points into one focal point and move the one subsequent focal point in the direction that focuses the image on the retina.

In general, a person who has myopia (nearsighted) has good near sight and poor distance sight. A person with hyperopia (far-sighted) has good far sight and poor near sight. A person with astigmatism has poor near and far sight. The part of the comprehensive eye exam that measures the smallest letter size (visual angle) seen at a specific far or near testing distance is called visual acuity. A visual acuity test measure of 20/20 means you can see the 20-size letter at the far test distance of 20 ft. (6 M) or near test distance of 16″ (40 cm). A visual acuity of 20/40 means you can see the 40-size letter (twice the size of the 20-size letter), and 20/200 means you can see the 200-size letter (ten times the size of the 20/20 size letter) at the testing distance. A visual acuity measure of 20/20 is considered normal. Physical refractive errors can be related to mental refractive errors by comparison learning.

Mental myopia is very much like myopia. In general, a person with myopia has good near vision and poor distance vision. A person with mental myopia also has good near vision and poor far vision but the measure of acuity is not in Ref. to the spatial domain (physical distance of 20 ft. or 16″) but rather in Ref. to the time domain (temporal dimensions of past, present, and future). Mental myopia may exist in various degrees but may present as preoccupation with present daily tasks and poor far strategic planning or the impulsive tendency of committing to an action without foresight to first considering the future consequences of the action in the present. Mental myopia could also present as good backward focusing ability (e.g., past trauma) and poor forward focusing ability (e.g., the ability to resolve past trauma and live in the present or plan). The person who has mental hyperopia would exhibit the opposite qualities like daydreaming or focusing on an anticipated event, considering the consequences of actions before committing to them, dissociation, and blocking out unresolved trauma. A person with mental astigmatism can manifest characteristics of a person with mental myopia and hyperopia.

Glaucoma is a medical eye condition that causes loss of peripheral (side) vision. Age-related macular degeneration (AMD) is a medical eye condition that causes loss of central vision. Geographic atrophy (GA) is the late-stage form of age-related macular degeneration. Cataract is a medical eye condition that causes loss of the full field of vision due to clouding of the transparent lens inside the eye. Strabismus is a medical eye condition where the two eyes are misaligned, causing the eye focusing and pointing mechanisms to have difficulty working together to point single point in space, creating double vision. The brain cannot process double images and may adapt by suppressing one image to avoid visual confusion. Suppression of vision may lead to amblyopia, the loss of vison.

Mental glaucoma, like glaucoma, affects the field of vision. With glaucoma, central vision is good but peripheral vision is poor. Likewise, mental glaucoma (MGlau) is a condition where there can be abnormal central focus on oneself, a selfish disposition, a bend toward narcissism and poor vision or concern for humanity and the benefit of others. It may also manifest somewhere on the spectrum of being introverted. Mental age-related macular degeneration (MAMD) is a condition also affecting visual field where a person may be so broadly and peripherally focused on the needs of others that they lose central sight of their own needs and neglect themselves. Mental cataracts (MCat) is a condition that can affect the full field of view where one may lose the overall ability to see and reason clearly. In extreme cases, MCat may lead to psychosis, hallucinations, and dissociation from reality. Mental strabismus (MStrab) is a condition that may manifest as a person with bipolar condition, manic-depression, schizophrenia, or multiple personality disorder where there is difficulty integrating and processing two or more different views of oneself or conflicting worldviews.

Mental optical illusions (MOil) are strange situations when things do not match up to reality. A mental optical illusion mirage may manifest as the false appearance of an oasis (person, place, or thing) or safe harbor that does not match up with reality. Mental illusion may also occur in the instance of mental diseases and disorders that can cause hallucinations, irrational thoughts, and unexpected, bizarre behavior. "Only by looking at an image from multiple viewpoints will one realize the true nature of the image ([6], p. 21)."

2.2.2 Spiritual pivot: spiritual vision

Learning by comparison is like mental gymnastics. It builds the strength and flexibility necessary to transition from one vantage point to another. Comparison learning helps one make the transition from physical optics to physiological optics, from physiological optics to physical refractive conditions, from physical refractive conditions to metaphysical mental refractive conditions, and from physical medical eye conditions to metaphysical mental medical eye conditions. Mental vision is the first type of metaphysical vision. Now we will pivot from physical vision to spiritual vision, the second type of metaphysical vision.

Pivoting to spiritual vision from mental vision is natural propagation and iteration. As with mental vision, spiritual vision uses comparison learning to switch back-and-forth from focusing on physical realities (physiological optics and medical eye conditions) to focusing on metaphysical realities (mental and psychological conditions and situations). The accommodative rock between the physical and the metaphysical creates mental flexibility, convictional strength, and is an important component of this metaphysical refraction. This process will allow us to bring into alignment and then converge into sharp focus relevant information from differing vantage points.

As a reminder, a person who has myopia (nearsighted) has good near sight and poor distance sight. A person with hyperopia (far-sighted) has good far sight and poor near sight. A person with astigmatism has poor near and far sight. The eye test that measures the smallest letter size (visual angle) seen at a far or near testing distance is called visual acuity. Whereas physical visual acuity is connected to a measurement in the spatial domain (e.g., 20 ft./6 M), you may recall that metaphysical mental visual acuity is connected to a measure in the temporal domain (past, present, and future). Spiritual visual acuity is also connected to the temporal domain but includes the extended ability to see from eternity to eternity, from before time (Ancient of days) to after time (end of days), and factor this sight into the decision-making process. In other words, spiritual acuity includes the ability to look at the origin of things and things that are eternal (See **Figure 3**, APVE spiritual vision visual acuity).

A person with spiritual myopia, just like the person with mental myopia, has good near sight and poor far sight but the measure of acuity extends to eternity. Spiritual myopia may present as preoccupation with temporal matters of physical life and poor focus on the eternal nature and destiny of the human soul and spirit. There may be an impulsive tendency to commit an action without first considering the eternal consequences of the action. Spiritual myopia could also present as a predominant focus on the hardship and struggles associated with daily life and poor distance focusing ability on faith-based hope that can empower one to survive and thrive in the heat of the day. Hope has the power to pull us forward through life's difficulties and lift us from depression and depravity to new heights in human technological achievement and wellness when focused on the fullness of life. The person who has spiritual hyperopia would exhibit the opposite qualities of spiritual myopia and could manifest as an extreme focus on eternal matters to the point of neglecting physical human needs, desires, and wants. The spiritual hyperopia may also consistently consider the eternal consequences of actions before committing to them. A person with spiritual astigmatism can manifest characteristics of a person with spiritual myopia and spiritual hyperopia.

As you may recall, glaucoma is a medical eye condition affecting the visual field causing loss of peripheral (side) vision, age-related macular degeneration causes loss of central vision, and a cataract can cause an overall loss of field of view. Strabismus is eye misalignment causing double vision that can lead to suppression of vision and loss of vision. Spiritual glaucoma (SGlau) is a condition where there is an abnormal field of view. With humanity as the fixation point, SGlau can manifest as a narcissistic viewpoint of oneself and the gradual loss of an overarching transcendent and mindful

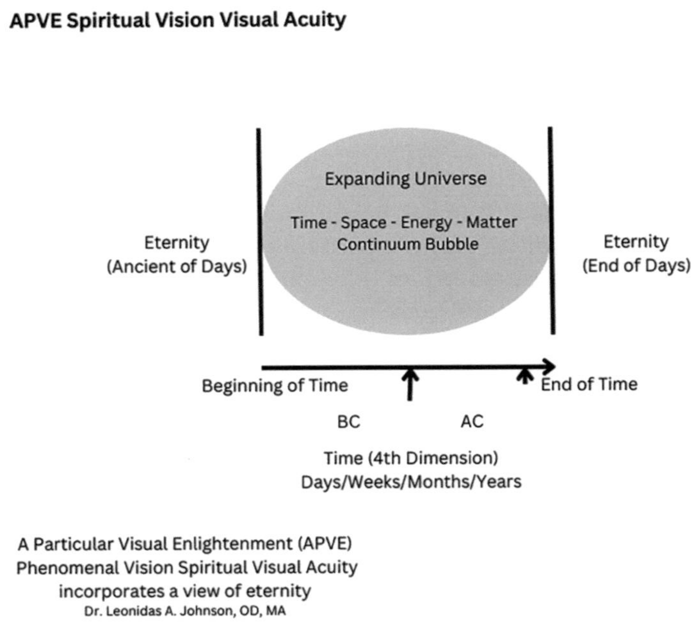

Figure 3.
APVE spiritual vision visual acuity.

view of God. God's presence is out of the field of view. Spiritual age-related macular degeneration (SAMD) is also a field of view disorder. With humanity as the fixation point, there is a gradual loss of vision of a narcissistic and egotistical view of oneself with a preserved humbling transcendent mindfulness view of God. God's presence remains in the field of view. Spiritual cataract (SCat) is a condition where there is a gradual loss, obstructed, hazy, or cloudy overarching view of God. Spiritual strabismus (SStrab) is a situation where the person may exhibit double vision, one heavenly (eternal) view and one earthly (perishable) view. Double vision causes visual confusion. The brain avoids visual confusion by suppressing one image. SStrab may manifest as someone struggling to make a decision to commit to science or religion/spirituality using linear deductive logic.

Spiritual optical illusion (SOil) is a strange, false, or deceptive situation where things do not match up with truth and reality. A spiritual optical illusion mirage may manifest as the false appearance of an oasis (person, place, or thing) or safe harbor that does not match up with reality. Spiritual illusions may also occur in situations involving witchcraft, dark magic, voodoo, false prophets, religious con artists, cults, satanic/demonic influences, and Reki (conduit of energy or spiritual entity).

2.3 Alignment and convergence of phenomenal vision (PVis) and three dimensions of human existence (TDoHE)

The physical, mental, and spiritual dimensions of vision are best understood when viewed through a lens that focuses on the trifold nature of human existence. The trifold nature or *Three Dimensions of Human Existence* (TDoHE) are *body, soul, and spirit*. The human body is physical in nature, mortal, and perishable. Upon death, the body deteriorates to the dust of the ground. The human body learns about the physical world through the five senses (e.g., sight, sound, smell, taste, and touch). The human soul is both physical and nonphysical in nature and is divisible into three parts, *emotions, mind, and volition*. Volition is also known as free-will or will-power. Some aspects of the human soul are mortal and some aspects are immortal. The human spirit is nonphysical in nature, is nonperishable, and immortal. Upon physical death, the human spirt continues to live in eternity. The human spirit is sensitive to supernatural entities and forces in the metaphysical world. According to the Bible, it is through the human spirit that humans can experience intimate fellowship with the Spirit of GOD.[1]

The three parts of the human soul are emotions, mind, and volition. Human emotions are influenced by the physical body and the physical world. The mind is influenced by the human spirit and the metaphysical world. The human mind is also impacted by a peculiar innate propensity and proclivity, within the human spirit, to call out and seek a relationship with God,[2] notable in times of danger or tragedy. The human soul is a bridge between the body and the spirit, between the physical and metaphysical. Upon a deeper inspection and dissection of the human soul, we can further see that volition is a fulcrum, a swivel, a hinge between human emotions and the human mind, between physical and metaphysical realities. Volition is a command center. *Human volition (will-power) is the emotional and mental process by which an individual human being decides on and commits to a specific course of action in life.*

Decisions may entail an element of uncertainty. Where there is uncertainty, there is room for hope and faith. Hope based on probability is reasonable but may not be expedient. Faith based on evidence that breeds confidence has value. Faith plays a role in mathematics, physics, astronomy, and the scientific method [9]. Faith has an emotional and mental component and impacts the decision-making process. The decision-making process is based on the concept of free-will. Free-will, according to the Bible, is evident in that God will not enter in the Human spirit unless invited.[3]

The alignment of Phenomenal Vision PVis with the Three Dimensions of Human Existence (TDoHE) can be seen when physical vision aligns with the human body, mental vision aligns with the human soul, and spiritual vision aligns with the human spirit. Physical vision is in the domain of the physical world, spiritual vision is in the domain of the metaphysical world, and mental vision is in both the physical and metaphysical domains. Three Dimensions of Human Existence (TDoHE) serves well as an aid in the discussion of metaphysical realities from a religious/spiritual and psychological perspective.

2.4 Pivot to traditional east Asian medicine (TEAM)

The concept of the Three Dimensions of Human Existence (TDoHE) can be correlated with holistic health and wellness theories of Traditional East Asian Medicine (TEAM).

> *Healing, however, is shaped not only by the clean lines of theory but also by the messy contingencies of practice; not only by doctors but also by complex interactions among physicians, patients, and nonphysicians caregivers: not only in the exclusive domain of*

[1] Refs. [7, 8] Rom 8:1-11.

[2] Refs. [7, 8] cf. Acts 17:24-27.

[3] Refs. [7, 8] cf. Rev. 3:19-20.

> *licensed doctors but also in the competition of diverse types of healers; not only in the crisis of illness but also in the day-to-day care of health and in the pursuit of salvation and enlightenment; not only by the exigencies of the sickroom but also by parameters negotiated in complex institutional and economic environments ([10], p. 1).*

The major philosophical foundations of Traditional East Asian Medicine (TEAM), sometimes referred to as Traditional Chinese Medicine (TCM) or Traditional Oriental Medicine (TOM), include Confucianism, Daoism, Naturalism, and Legalism originating from China and Buddhism originating from India.

Acupuncture is one of the four pillars of Traditional East Asian Medicine (alongside Tui Na, Herbal Medicine, and Qi Gong) [11]. Tui Na should not be viewed as a massage or a bodywork therapy, but rather as a whole medical system that can be used to treat the whole body for both external and internal conditions ([12], p. 19). Qigong involves using exercises to optimize energy within the body, mind, and spirit, with the goal of improving and maintaining health and well-being [13]. The four pillars/disciplines of Traditional East Asian Medicine (TEAM) use different methods to influence qi for health and well-being.

The practice of Traditional East Asian Medicine (TEAM) is based on the movement of qi in the body through the channel network (jing luo). There are at least six channel layers. The most superficial channel layer is the cutaneous regions, followed by the sinew channels, the luo vessels, the primary channels, the divergent channels, and the deepest level, the extraordinary vessels. The channel network functions to transport qi and blood throughout the body and render the body as an integrated whole, protect the body by serving as a series of barriers to prevent the deeper penetration of pathogenic factors from the exterior, respond to dysfunction in the body, and to transmit qi to organs and areas allowing for the healing process to occur [14]. Scientific research in acupuncture has grown exponentially in the past 20 years. Acupuncture enjoys a high level of clinical evidence for dozens of conditions and is one of the most widely recommended treatments in modern medicine [15].

2.5 Alignment and convergence of phenomenal vision (PVis), three dimensions of human existence (TDoHE), and Yin-Yang theory (YY-theory)

The philosophy of Traditional East Asian Medicine (TEAM) philosophy rests on the foundation of the Yin-Yang Theory (YY-Theory) and Five-Phase Correspondence Theory (FP-Theory).

> *The theory of yin and yang, derived from agelong observations of nature, describes the way phenomena naturally group in pairs of opposites – heaven and earth, sun and moon, night and day, winter, and summer, male and female, up and down, inside, and outside, movement and stasis." ([16–18], p. 1).*

> *The Chinese characters for 'Yin' and 'Yang' are related to the image of a hill with one side dark and the other sunlit....Thus the character for Yin indicates the shady side of a hill, whilst the character for Yang indicates the sunny side of a hill. By extension, they therefore also indicate 'darkness' and 'light' or 'shady' and 'bright' ([19, 20], p. 4).*

The concept of yin and yang (YY-Theory) aligns with the concept of Three Dimensions of Human Existence (TDoHE) in the following manner, the body aligns with yin, the soul aligns with both yin and yang, and the human spirit aligns with yang. Upon further dissection of the soul, human emotion aligns with yin and yang but more yin, the mind aligns with yin and yang but more yang, and volition aligns with both yin and yang equally when balanced (see *APVE Engendering and Restraining Cycle illustration*).

The concept of the "Three Treasures" (Ling/Essence, Qi, and Shen/soul/spirit) also aligns with the concept of the Three Dimensions of Human Existence (TDoHE) where the human body corresponds to the yin nature of Ling/Essence, the soul corresponds to the yin/yang nature of Qi, and the human spirit corresponds to the yang nature of Shen (soul/spirit). Another way yin yang theory (YY-Theory) aligns with the concept of Three Dimensions of Human Existence (TDoHE) is to align the cosmological concept of heaven as the yang element, earth as the yin element, and humans as a yin/yang connecting element, humanity as a pillar that connects heaven (yang) to earth (yin). In this alignment, humanity can be viewed as the pivot between physical and metaphysical realities (see *APVE Chart Illustration*).

2.5.1 Sample APVE pattern diagnosis: APVE Yang vacuity

If a direct spiritual relationship between the human spirit and the Spirit of God is absent in terms of Three Dimensions of Human Existence (TDoHE), then in terms of Traditional East Asian Medicine (TEAM), this would represent an identifiable and distinct diagnosis pattern.

> *Pattern differentiation is the process by which clinical information (obtained from the examination) is analyzed, synthesized, and inferred, leading to a clear representation of a particular phase of a disease in a TCM (traditional Chinese medicine) pattern. Pattern (zheng) is a combination of signs and/or symptoms that forms a distinct clinical picture indicative of a particular disorder ([21], p. 4).*

The absence of a direct spiritual connection between the human spirit and the Spirit of God in terms of Three Dimensions of Human Existence (TDoHE) thought would correspond to a *APVE Yang Vacuity (Deficiency)* pattern in Traditional East Asian Medicine (TEAM) thought. This type of deficiency would prevent one from obtaining the fullness of life experience.

2.6 Alignment of phenomenal vision (PVis), three dimensions of human existence (TDoHE), Yin and Yang theory (YY-theory), and five-phase theory (FP-theory)

The five-Phase theory of correspondence (FP-Theory) is an extension of Yin and Yang Theory (YY-Theory). The five-phase theory (FP-Theory) follows the belief that the human body is subject to and corresponds with a five-phase cause-and-effect relationship that governs the universe.

> *The theory of the five phases rests on the notion that all phenomena in the universe are the products of the movement and mutation of five qualities: wood, fire, earth, metal, and water ([16–18], p. 7).*

> *The Illustrated Supplement to the Categorized Canon (lei jing tu yi) states: "The dynamic of Creation cannot be without engendering or restraining; without*

engendering there is no way by which things may arise, and without restraining, things become unduly powerful and cause harm." ([16–18], pp. 8, 9).

Five-phase theory (FP-Theory) is used not only to diagnose and treat the human body and internal organs (aka zang/fu organs) but also the soul/spirit. Wood corresponds to the liver and gall bladder. Fire corresponds to the heart/pericardium and small intestine/san jiao. Earth corresponds to the spleen and stomach. Metal corresponds to the lung and large intestine. Water corresponds to the kidney and urinary bladder.

Concepts of the human spirit and soul are entangled in the five-phase correspondence theory ([19, 20], pp. 99, 100). In a broad sense, the spirit describes the total external manifestation of vital activities which reflect the functions of the zang/fu organs, and in a narrow sense, it describes mental actives including consciousness and cognitive activities ([21], pp. 11, 12). Observation of the spirt plays a key role in TCM diagnosis ([21], p. 14).

There is no distinction between the human soul and the human spirit in Traditional East Asian Medicine (TEAM). The combined concept of soul/spirit is referred to as Shen (Shen spelled with a capital "S"). Shen with capital "S" is distinguished from shen with a small "s." Shen with capital "S" represents the overall concept of soul/spirit and shen with small "s" represents the five-phase aspect of soul/spirit which most closely corresponds to the emotional aspects of the mind.

Shen is further subdivided into the following five aspects with respect to five-phase theory:

1. Wood = Ethereal soul/spirit (Hun)

2. Fire = shen soul/spirit (shen spelled with a small "s")

3. Earth = Intellect soul/spirit (Yi)

4. Metal = Corporeal soul/spirit (Po)

5. Water = Will-power soul/spirit (Zhi) ([19, 20], pp. 99, 100).

The Five-phase correspondence Theory (FP-Theory) aligns with the concept of the Three Dimensions of Human Existence (TDoHE) in the following manner: the *Body* of TDoHE corresponds to *Po* (corporal soul/spirit) and is the Metal phase of FP-Theory, the *Emotion* component of the human Soul of TDoHE corresponds to *shen* (mind/emotion soul/spirit) and is the Fire phase, the *Mind* component of the human Soul corresponds to *Yi* (intellect soul/spirit) and is the Earth phase, and the *Volition* component of the human Soul corresponds to *Zhi* (will-power soul/spirit) and is the Water phase of FP-Theory, and the *Human Spirit* of TDoHE corresponds to *Hum* (Ethereal soul/spirit) and is the Wood phase of FP-Theory (see **Figure 1**, i.e., APVE FOL, APVE Graphic, and **Figure 4**, i.e., APVE Engendering and Restraining illustrations).

2.6.1 Sample APVE pattern diagnosis: APVE ethereal/wood deficiency pattern

If a direct spiritual relationship between the human spirit and the Spirit of God is absent in terms of Three Dimensions of Human Existence (TDoHE), this condition would be identified as an *APVE Ethereal/Wood Deficiency Pattern*. It is a religious/spiritual pattern that can have multiple physical and psychosocial manifestations.

DOI: http://dx.doi.org/10.5772/intechopen.1006067

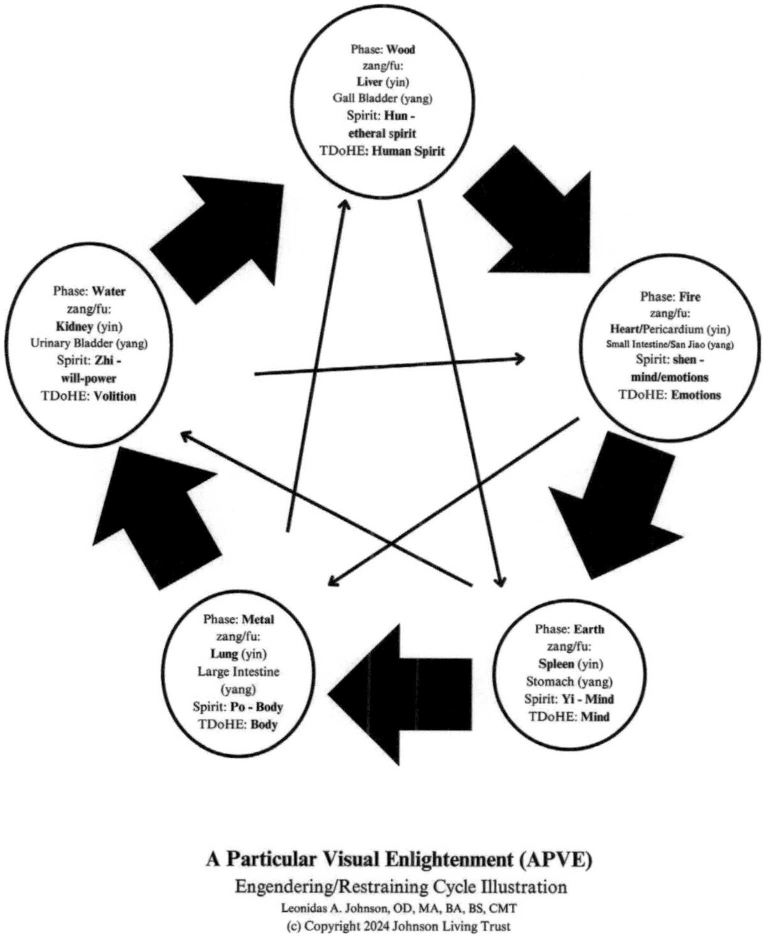

Figure 4.
APVE engendering and restraining illustration.

The *Ethereal Wood Deficiency Pattern* can be described as a failure of Water/Zhi (i.e., Human Soul-Volition) to engender Wood/Hum (i.e., Human Spirit) in the engendering cycle (Sheng cycle) and an excess or overwhelming of Metal/Po (i.e., Human Body) over Wood/Hum (i.e., Human Spirit) in the restraining cycle (Ke cycle). This could also result in a failure of Wood/Hum (i.e., Human Spirit) to restrain Earth/Yi (i.e., Human Soul-Mind) in the restraining cycle causing Earth/Yi (i.e., Human Soul-Mind) to rebel against Wood/Hum (i.e., Human Spirit) in the restraining cycle and further excess of Metal (Body) from Earth (Soul-Mind) in the engendering cycle.

When the human emotional and mental decision-making process is unbalanced, various metaphysical (psychological, psychosocial, spiritual) and physical (psychosomatic, structural, functional, sensory) dysfunctions may follow.

2.7 Energy medicine

There are two important aspects of Traditional East Asian Medicine (TEAM), the first has to do with vital energy or qi. Health is a result of the proper balance (yin/yang) of vital energy (qi) in the body, and disease is a result of imbalance ([22, 23], p. 17). According to Traditional East Asian Medicine, qi, blood, essence, and fluids are the basic elements of all physiological activity.

> *Blood and fluids are the sustenance of the body, nourishing and moistening the entire organism, and are yin in nature. Essence is the basis of physical development and reproduction. It is the store surplus potential of the human body, and the basis and fluid production. All changes that occur in the human body from birth to death result from the interaction of qi, blood, essence, and fluids.*
>
> *The word "qi" originally meant cloud or mist. Ancient Chinese natural philosophers, observing how clouds and mist gathered and dispersed, lighted on the idea that the whole universe was made of one basic substance, qi, that could assume many different forms. They also posited that a formless, invisible, diffuse, and active form of qi was responsible for all movement and change in the universe. ([16–18], p. 17).*

Qi is the basis for all physiological and emotional activities of the body. In Traditional East Asian Medicine (TEAM), the Wood phase and Liver zang/fu organ greatly impact emotions.

> *"...emotional activity is closely related to the liver qi. Only when the function of the liver in maintaining the free flow of qi is normal can the qi and blood be harmonious and the mind at ease. Dysfunction of the liver, therefore, is often accompanied by emotional changes such as mental depression or excitement. When liver qi stagnates, for example, there may be mental depression, paranoia, or even weeping; when the liver qi is hyperactive, there may be irascibility, insomnia, dream disturbed sleep, dizziness and vertigo. While dysfunction of the liver often leads to emotional changes, at the same time prolonged excessive mental irritation often leads to dysfunction of the liver in maintaining the free flow of qi. ([24], p. 36).*
>
> *Liver-Blood and Liver-Qi need to be harmonized and Liver-Blood must root Liver-Qi to prevent its becoming stagnant or rebelling upwards....The Spiritual Axis in Chapter 8 says, "If the Liver is deficient there will be fear; if it is in excess there will be ager." ([25], p. 33).*

Dalton's Atomic Theory postulates that all matter is composed of atoms. Even though we now know that the atom is divisible to a nucleus consisting of positively charged protons, neutral charge neutrons, and orbiting negatively charged electrons, Dalton's theory is still largely true. The human body, which consists of 45–75% water molecules by mass [26], consists of atoms, vibrating, in constant motion. It is no wonder that the human body emits an energy field (biofield). This can explain why the human body is receptive to various forms of energy including the electromagnetic (EM) fields of other humans.

> *Inside the body is a living matrix of connective tissue fabric consisting of fascia, extracellular matrices, integrins, cytoskeletons, nuclear matrices, and DNA, governed by tensegrity, subject to entrainment, that generates piezobioeletric signals, carries bioelectric signals between every part of the body, and maintains electrical homeostasis throughout the body ([1], p. 588).*

Increasing knowledge of the living matrix of the human body, tensegrity [27], entrainment [28], human biological rhythms [29], the role of the practitioner's heart in health care [30], the human biofield [31], and biological aspects of physics continue to give birth to new complementary therapies. Biological aspects of physics contributing to ingenuity in health and wellness include motion (linear, rotational, gravity), vibration (waves, sound, light) electricity, magnetism, hydrodynamics, thermodynamics, and heart coherence. Promising new health-oriented therapies are numerous and include sound therapy [32], music therapy [33, 34], music medicine [35], meditation [36], prayer [37], reiki [38], therapeutic touch [39], earthing (grounding) [40], electromagnetic radiation (EMR) therapies in the visible [41] and infrared (IR) [42] spectrums, and extracorporeal shock wave therapy [43].

> *Current knowledge about the roles of electrical, magnetic, elastic, acoustic, thermal, gravitational, and photonic energies in living systems shows that most likely no single "life force" or "healing energy" exist. Rather, the living body seems to have many energy systems, and there seem to be many ways of influencing those systems ([1], p. 589).*

The salutogenic spectrum of wellness from the vantage points of Traditional East Asian Medicine (TEAM), Western allopathic medicine, and Energy Medicine can all be aligned and converged to create a depth of focus that puts the focal point image of the fullness of life in clear view (see **Table 1**, i.e., APVE Chart Illustrations and **Figure 1**, i.e., APVE Eye Graphic).

2.8 Refracting the physical metaphysical pendulum

There are two important aspects of Traditional East Asian Medicine (TEAM), the first has to do with vital energy or qi. The second important aspect of Traditional East Asian Medicine (TEAM) has to do with its celestial origin.

> *Knowledge of these medical modalities is divinely revealed to humans from celestial sources,...every major aspect of Chinese medicine had is origin attributed to the writings and teachings of semi-mythical divine rulers in the line of Chinese Emperors, attribution to the heavens as the source of all human knowledge, which is channeled through demigod rulers, to mortal humans, forms the basis for Chinese civilization in general, as well as for health and healing ([23], p. 18).*

The record of this spiritual origin is found in the Huang Di Nei Jing.

> *"Huang Di Nei Jing 《黄帝内经》 Yellow Emperor's Inner Canon) is the earliest and most important written work of Traditional Chinese Medicine. It was compiled over 2200 years ago during the Warring States period (475–221 BC) and is regarded as the fundamental and most representative medical text. The version nominated for inscription in the Memory of the World Register was printed and published by Hu's Gulin Sanctum in 1339 using the woodblock-printing technique. It is the earliest and the best-preserved version of its kind now extant."* [4]

[4] silkroads@UNESCO.org, 2022.

Phenomenal vision (PVis)	Three dimensions of human existence TDoHE	Yin-Yang theory YY-theory	Three treasures	Cosmology heaven earth pillar	Five-phase correspondence theory FP-theory	Energy medicine
Physical vision	**BODY** (Human) Nature: Mortal Antenna sensitivity: Physical receptor	Yin	Yin (Ling/Essence)	Yin (Earth)	Phase: **METAL** ZangFu: Lung/Large intestines Shen (spirit/soul): Po (Corporeal)	Human Biofield(s) (e.g., Heart EM Field)
Mental vision	**SOUL** (Emotions) Nature: Mortal + Immortal Antenna sensitivity: Physical + Nonphysical Metaphysical receptor	Yin & Yang Yin > Yang	Yin & Yang (Qi)	Yin & Yang (Humanity)	Phase: **FIRE** ZangFu: Heart/Small intestine Pericardium/San Jiao Shen (spirit/soul): shen (mind/emotions)	Human Biofield(s) (e.g., Heart EM Field)
Mental vision	**SOUL** (Volition/Will) Nature: Mortal + Immortal Antenna sensitivity: Physical + Nonphysical Metaphysical receptor	Yin & Yang Yin = Yang	Yin & Yang (Qi)	Yin & Yang (Humanity)	Phase: **WATER** ZangFu: Kidney/Urinary bladder Shen (spirit/soul): Zhi (will-power)	Human Biofield(s) (e.g., Heart EM Field)
Mental vision	**SOUL** (Mind) Nature: Mortal + Immortal Antenna sensitivity: Physical + Nonphysical Metaphysical receptor	Yin & Yang Yang> Yin	Yin & Yang (Qi)	Yin & Yang (Humanity)	Phase: **EARTH** ZangFu: Spleen/Stomach Shen (spirit/soul): Yi (mind)	Human Biofield(s) (e.g., Heart EM Field)
Spiritual vision	**SPIRIT** (Human) Nature: Immortal Antenna sensitivity: Nonphysical/Spirituality Energy + Entity receptor	Yang	Yang (Shen)	Yang (Heavens)	Phase: **WOOD** ZangFu: Liver/Gallbladder Shen (spirit/soul): (Hun) Ethereal soul (eternal)	• 7 Auric Layers • 7 Chakra • Energy Centers • Reiki • Energy/Qi Gong acupuncture etc.

Table 1.
A Particular Visual Enlightenment (APVE) chart illustration.

> *Over time, the Inner Canon has been rearranged by editors into three sections, forming separate books: The Basic Questions (Su Wen), The Numinous/Spiritual Pivot (Ling Shu), and the Grand Basis (Taisu). Taken together, they discuss acupuncture, the piercing of the body with stones and needles in order to influence the qi, and moxibustion, heat treatment to the same end, often performed by burning the plant called mugwort." ([10], p. 35).*

The Huang Di Nei Jing Ling Shu (aka the *Spiritual Pivot* or *Spiritual Axis*) shines a light on the spiritual foundation of the healing arts.

> *"All norms of piercing [require one] to first of all consider the spirit as the foundation." [44].*

> *...the Jin Yue Quan Shu says: 'Adeptness at understanding the meaning of the spirit [is essential]. It is the root of life and death, it cannot be investigated.' ([45], p. 4).*

The notion that the spirit is the root of life and death is not novel. According to the Bible, spiritual sickness and death preceded physical sickness and death. The Christian Bible continues to be, "the best-selling book of all time," [46] claiming to be the revelation of God the creator of the universe, and the source of all answers to metaphysical questions concerning the origin of things, things that are eternal, and purpose of life. The genesis of human sickness is found in the story of Adam and Eve, part of the creation narrative, in the third chapter of the book of Genesis.[5] The Bible also shines a light on the spiritual foundation for healing.[6]

The importance of religious and spiritual beliefs and practices in health and well-being has great significance in the practice of all forms of modern evidence-based medicine. The importance of religion/spirituality has been downplayed, overlooked, and discouraged at various times and in various ways around the world. The primary reasoning used in science is Aristotelian linear deductive logic where two opposites cannot be true. The primary reasoning used in religion/spirituality and Traditional East Asian Medicine (TEAM) is inductive logic that is complimentary of opposites (e.g., YY-Theory). Inductive logic is a more circular, sexier, logic in that it swerves and curves. Light, is it a wave or a particle? According to deductive linear logic, it presents a paradox, an oxymoron, it can only be one or the other but not both. According to inductive logic, it can be and is both, opposites can be true. Translogical ([9], p. 25; [47], p. 30) thinking embraces paradoxical truths. Deductive and inductive logic may have the same final destination, but the journey is different. The push to advance innovation and modern technology in medicine via scientific methodology has been, at times, accompanied by a counter push to separate and distance advances in medicine via religion/spirituality methods, in both Eastern (separation from shamanism) [10] and Western medicine (separation model in which medicine neglects and avoids spirituality/religion) [48, 49].

The pendulum between science and religion/spirituality has started to swing the other way. Recently, the pendulum between physical and metaphysical health realities has swung toward an explosive growth and acceptance in the number of peer-reviewed articles on the impact of religion/spirituality in medicine ([50–52], p. 3; [53], p. 435). The relationship between science and religion/spirituality is

---

[5] Refs. [7, 8] Gen. 3:1-24.

[6] Refs. [7, 8] John 3:16; John 10:10.

becoming more complementary, especially when the focus is on issues that build bridges, like wellness and fullness of life, and less adversarial when the focus is on issues that build walls. There is a wealth of evidence supporting the impact religion/spirituality has on wound healing, surgical recovery, overall health, well-being ([54], p. 1225; [55], p. 7; [56], p. 1) including now the impact on the human biofield [57]. As a result, 90% of US medical schools now include academic curricula that include courses that focus on the impact of religion and spirituality on health and well-being ([50–52], pp. 9–10; [58]). It is with this progressive understanding that the World Health Organization defines health as a state of complete physical, mental, and social well-being and not merely the absence of disease or infirmity [59].

The alignment and convergence of science and religion, deductive and inductive reasoning, Western allopathic medicine and Traditional East Asian Medicine (TEAM), and health and wellness can be but need not be problematic. The pendular swing between science and religion, between allopathic and alternative medicine can be likened to a refraction of physical and metaphysical realities. Looking at one image of reality, then switching to a different image of reality, always comparing the clarity of one image to the other, and making necessary adjustments along the way until both images are equally clear is a type of metaphysical Jackson cross-cylinder (JCC) [60, 61] refraction. It is possible, through a process called metaphysical refraction, to bring the images of Western medicine, traditional East Asian medicine (TEAM), energy medicine, alternative medicine, and religion/spirituality into clearer focus by not just converging them to a salutogenic depth of focus but rather to a centered focal point image of the fullness of life. A biopsychosocial-spiritual model is blooming in Western Medicine where the biologic, social, psychologic, and spiritual aspects of the person are seen as being inextricably linked with each other ([62], p. 655; [63], p. 352). The APVE refractive tool is simply the inquiry about physical, mental, and spiritual vision during a patient's initial intake or follow-up encounter along with the use of the APVE diagrams. The APVE tool guides the encounter into a holistic biopsychosocial-spiritual model of care, a Western version of TEAM.

The alignment and convergence of Phenomenal Vision (PVis) (i.e., the life-changing ability to take a general understanding of physical vision and compare that understanding to mental and spiritual vision) and Three Dimensions of Human Existence (TDoHE – i.e., the human consists of a body, soul, and spirit where the soul further consists of emotions, mind, and volition) and concepts of Yin-Yang (YY-Theory) and Five-Phase Correspondence Theory (FP-Theory) of Traditional East Asian Medicine (TEAM) is somewhat reminiscent of preparing a delicious serving of New Orleans seafood gumbo. Ingredients of New Orleans gumbo may include blue crab, shrimp, andouille sausage, smoked turkey meat, chicken meat, green bell pepper, red onions, celery, fresh okra, and various other spices and creole seasonings (see **Figure 2**, i.e., APVE FOL illustration). Now for the finishing touch, a sprinkle of gumbo file (ground sassafras leaves), the cause-and-effect paradigm.

2.9 Universal cause-effect paradigm

The final step in this refraction of physical and metaphysical realities includes the use of a paradigm prism to balance cause-and-effect phenomena.

2.9.1 APVE universal cause-and-effect paradigm

1. The Paradigm of Cause-and Effect Relations between Correspondence Phenomena

    1.1. Causation through Mysterious & Magical Correspondence

    1.1.1. Physical Laws

    1.1.1.1. Known & Explainable Physical Laws (e.g., science of physics, astronomy, and mathematics)

    1.1.1.1.1. Only 5% of the observable universe is visible to humans.

    1.1.1.2. Unknown & Unexplainable Physical Laws

    1.1.1.2.1. 95% of the observable universe is invisible to us and beyond it is an unobservable universe that is 100% invisible to us ([9], pp. 8, 15).

    1.1.2. Contact Phenomena

    1.1.2.1. Contact or former union between two elements creates a relationship in which a manipulation of one of the elements produces a visible effect upon the other although separated by distance (e.g., Voodoo doll).

    1.1.3. Homeopathic (contagious/noncontagious) Phenomena

    1.1.3.1. Like corresponds to like. Harm inflicted on the image of a person results in harm to the person although separated by distance. May also include the concept of vibrational correspondence grossly alluded to in Hidden Messages in Water [64].

    1.2. Causation through Systematic Correspondence

    1.2.1. Yin-Yang Correspondence Theory

    1.2.2. Five-Phases Correspondence Theory

2. The Paradigm of Cause-and-Effect Relations between Noncorresponding Phenomena

    2.1. Causation through Influence of Natural Phenomena (*Physical Vision*)

    2.1.1. Non-infectious

    2.1.2. Infectious

2.2. Causation through Influence of Mental/Social Phenomena (*Mental Vision*)

2.2.1. Psychological

2.2.2. Psychosomatic

2.2.3. Socioeconomical political (e.g., Hegemony)

2.3. Causation through Influence of Supranatural (unexplained) Phenomena – Miraculous Signs and Wonders (*Spiritual Vision*)

2.3.1. GOD (exist outside the time-space-energy-matter bubble)

2.3.2. Metaphysical Biblical Laws

2.3.2.1. Example:

2.3.2.1.1. Law of sin and death [7, 8] Ez. 18:4; Rom. 3:23

2.3.2.1.2. The Gospel Message [7, 8] John 3:16; Rom. 6:23

2.3.3. Spirit beings

2.3.3.1. Angelic

2.3.3.2. Satanic

2.3.3.3. Ancestral

3. Conclusion

A Particular Visual Enlightenment (APVE) is a metaphysical refraction, and as a tool, can be used as a corrective lens to see health and wellness more clearly from a physical, mental, and spiritual point of view. It brings into focus bridges that connect Eastern and Western Health philosophies. It increases cultural religious/spiritual sensitivity and competence in clinical practice. Simply asking the patient about their physical, mental, and spiritual vision during the subjective intake serves as a natural guide into discussions about mental health (mental vision) and their religious/spiritual health and engagement in life (spiritual vision). It clarifies the emotional and mental dynamics at play in the decision-making process. It offers a foundation for the development of a personal decision-making strategy for difficult life decisions. It reinforces holistic interprofessional communication. It breaks down barriers between science and religion, deductive (Aristotelian linear logic) and inductive reasoning (logic that swerves and curves), Western allopathic medicine and Traditional East Asian Medicine (TEAM), and promotes alternative therapies, complementary therapies, integrative medicine, and energy medicine.

Life's greatest disease is death. On the other end of the spectrum is the fullness of life. The ministry of healing is a high calling; therefore, healers must always adhere to a high standard. *A Particular Visual Enlightenment,* when used as a corrective lens, can help the healer stretch toward the mark and high calling by bringing into clear focus an image of the fullness of life.

APVE diagrams and illustrations

See **Figures 1–4** and **Table 1**.

Conflict of interest

The author declares no conflict of interest.

Acronyms and abbreviations

TEAM	traditional East Asian medicine
APVE	a particular visual enlightenment
BVA	best visual acuity
DOF	depth of focus
FOL	fullness of life
PVis	phenomenal vision
TDoHE	three dimensions of human existence
YY-theory	Yin-Yang theory
FP-theory	five-phase theory
UCEP	universal cause-effect paradigm
AOD	ancient of days
AMD	age-related macular degeneration
GA	geographic atrophy
MGlau	mental glaucoma
MAMD	mental age-related macular degeneration
MCat	mental cataracts
MStrab	mental strabismus
MOil	mental optical illusion
SGlau	spiritual glaucoma
SAMD	spiritual age-elated macular degeneration
SCat	spiritual cataracts
SStrab	spiritual strabismus
SOil	spiritual optical illusion
EM	electromagnetic
EMR	electromagnetic radiation
IR	infrared EM
JCC	Jackson cross-cylinder

Author details

Leonidas A. Johnson[1,2]

1 Midwestern University Chicago College of Optometry, Downers Grove, Illinois, United States of America

2 Pacific College of Health and Science, Chicago, Illinois, United States of America

*Address all correspondence to: leonidasjohnson@hotmail.com

References

[1] Fritz S, Fritz LA. Fundamentals of Therapeutic Massage. 7th ed. St Louis: Elsevier; 2021

[2] Mittelmark MB, Bauer GF. Salutogenesis as a theory, as an orientation and as the sense of coherence. In: Mittelmark MB, Bauer GF, Vaandrager L, Pelikan JM, Eriksson M, Lindstrom B, Magistretti CM, editors. The Handbook of Salutogensis. 2nd ed. Cham: Springer; 2022. pp. 11-17. DOI: 10.1007/978-3-030-79515-3_3

[3] Rittle-Johnson B, Star JR. Chapter seven - The power of comparison in learning and instruction: Learning outcomes supported by different type of comparisons. In: Mestre JP, Ross BH, editors. Psychology of Learning and Motivation. Vol. 55. Academic Press; 2011. pp. 199-225. Available from: https://www.sciencedirect.com/science/article/pii/B9780123876911000077

[4] Krum R. Cool Infographics Effective Communication with Data Visualization and Design. Indianapolis: John Wiley & Sons, Inc.; 2014

[5] Gould S. How Eyesight Interlinks with Cognition: Advanced Vision Care from the Retina through the Brain. Elkins Park, PA: Salus University Center for Continuing and Post Graduate Education; 2021

[6] Johnson LA. Phenomenal Vision Eyesight to Life Sight. Meadville: Christian Faith Publishing, Inc; 2020

[7] Radmacher ED, Allen RB, House HW, editors. The NKJV Study Bible. 2nd ed. 2007

[8] Radmacher ED, Allen RB, House HW, editors. The NKJV Study Bible. 1997

[9] Guillen M. Believing Is Seeing a Physicist Explains How Science Shattered his Atheism and Revealed the Necessity of Faith. Carol Stream: Tyndale House Publishers; 2021

[10] Hinrichs TJ, Barnes LL. In: Hinrichs TJ, Barnes LL, editors. Chinese Medicine and Healing. Cambridge: The Belknap Press of Harvard University Press; 2013

[11] Busch S. Tui Na Hand Techniques - Pacific College of Health and Science BT130.71.2022F.CH. Lecture 1 Slide Deck. Chicago, IL, USA; 12 Sep 2022

[12] Aspell R. The Practice of Tui Na Principles, Diagnostics and Working with the Sinew Channels. London: Singing Dragon; 2019

[13] (NIH), NCCIH and the National Institutes of Health. Qigong: What You Need To Know. Bethesda, Maryland, USA; Feb 2022. Retrieved from National Center of Complemenatry and Integrative Health National Institutes of Health. Available from: https://www.nccih.nih.gov/health/qigong-what-you-need-to-know#:~:text=Qigong%2C%20pronounced%20%E2%80%9Cchi%20gong%2C,maintaining%20health%20and%20well%2Dbeing

[14] Collin MF. Aucpuncture Channels and Points 1 - Pacific College of Health and Science AC504A.71.2022F.CH. Lecture Slide Deck - Channel Layers and Functions. Chicago, IL, USA; Sep 2022

[15] Koppelman MH. Evidence Based Acupuncture: An Overview of Scientific Evidence. 1st ed. Barrington, Rhode Island, United States: Evidence Based Acupuncture; 2018. Employer Identification Number (EIN):

82-2078725. Available from: https://www.evidencebasedacupuncture.org/about-us/

[16] Wiseman N, Ellis A. Fundamentals of Chinese Medicine Revised Edition (Third Revised Edition Zhong Yi Ji Chu Xue). Taos New Mexico: Paradigm Publications; 1996

[17] Wiseman N, Ellis A. Fundamentals of Chinese Medicine Revised Edition (Third Revised Edition Zhong Yi Ji Chu Xue). Taos New Mexico: Paradigm Publications; 2015

[18] Wiseman N, Ellis A. Fundamentals of Chinese Medicine Revised Edition (Third Revised Edition Zhong Yi Ji Chu Xue). Taos New Mexico: Paradigm Publications; 2017

[19] Maciocia G. The Foundations of Chinese Medicine a Comprehensive Text for Acupuncturists and Herbalists. London: Churchill Livingstone Elsevier; 1989

[20] Maciocia G. The Foundations of Chinese Medicine a Comprehensive Text for Acupuncturists and Herbalists. London: Churchill Livingstone Elsevier; 2005

[21] Yi Q, Stone A. Traditional Chinese Medicine Diagnosis Study Guide. Seattle: Eastland Press, Inc; 2008

[22] Chen X, Cui J, Li R, Norton R, Park J, Kong J, et al. Dao yin (a.k.a. qigong): Origin, development, potential mechanisms, and clinical applications. Evidence-based Complementary and Alternative Medicine. 2019;**2019**(1):3705120. DOI: 10.1155/2019/3705120

[23] Micozzi MS. Celestial Healing. London: Singing Drago; 2011

[24] Xinnong C, editor. Chinese Acupuncture and Moxibustion. 4th ed. (X. Zhufan, L. Yachan, X. Yao, L. Xiaozhen, & W. Huizhu, Trans.). Beijing, People's Republic of China: Foreign Languages Press; 2019

[25] Maciocia G. The Psyche in Chinese Medicine Treatment of Emotional and Mental Disharmonies with Acupuncture and Chinese Herbs. Great Britain: Elsevier; 2009

[26] Zhang J, Zhang N, Du S, Liu S, Ma G. Acute water supplementation improved the body composition of young female adults after water restriction of 12h in Baoding, China: A randomized controlled trial (RCT). Frontiers in Nutrition. 2022;**9**:880630. DOI: 10.3389/fnut.2022.880630

[27] Ingber DE. From tensegrity to human organs-on-chips: Implications for mechanobiology and mechanotherapeutics. Biochemical Journal. 2023;**480**(4):243-257. DOI: 10.1042/BCJ20220303

[28] Ingendoh RM, Posny ES, Heine A. Binaural beats to entrain the brain? A systematic review of the effects of binaural beat stimulation on brian oscillatory activity, and the implications for psychological research and intervention. PLoS One. 2023;**18**(5):e0286023. DOI: 10.1371/journal.pone.0286023

[29] Farhud D, Aryan Z. Circadian rhythm, lifestyle and health: A narrative review. Iranian Journal of Public Health. 2018;**47**:1068-1076

[30] Espinosa S. The therapeutic role of the practioner's heart in classical Chinese medicine and modern medical science. The European Journal of Oriental Medicine. 2014;**7**(5):18-25

[31] Hammerschlag R, Sprengel M, Baldwin AL. Biofield therapies: Guidelines for reporting clinical trials. Global Advances in Integrative Medicine and Health. 2024;**13**. DOI: 10.1177/27536130231202501. ISSN: 2753-6130, Online ISSN: 2753-6130

[32] Goldsby TL, Goldsby ME, McWalters M, Mills PJ. Sound healing: Mood, emotional, and spiritual well-being interrelationships. Religions. 2022;**13**(2):123. DOI: 10.3390/rel13020123

[33] DeWitte M, Pinho AD, Stams G-J, Moonen X, Bos AE, VanHooren S. Music therapy for stress reduction: A systematic review and meta-analysis. Health Psychology Review. 2022;**16**:134-159. DOI: 10.1080/17437199.2020.1846580

[34] Li K, Weng L, Wang X. The state of music therapy studies in the past 20 years: A bibliometric analysis. Frontiers in Psychology. 2021;**12**:697726. DOI: 10.3389/fpsyg.2021.697726

[35] Bleibel M, Cheikh AE, Sadier NS, Abou-Abbas L. The effect of music therapy on cognitive functions in patients with Alzheimer's disease: A systemic review of randomized controlled trials. Alzheimer's Research & Thearpy. 2023;**15**(1):65. DOI: 10.1186/s13195-023-01214-9

[36] Cearns M, Clark SR. The effects of dose, practice habits, and objects of focus on digital meditation effectiveness and adherence: Longitudinal study of 280,000 digital meditation sessions across 103 countries. Journal of Medical Internet Research. 2023;**25**:e43358. DOI: 10.2196/43358

[37] Upenieks L. Unpacking the relationship between prayer and anxiety: A consideration of prayer types and expectations in the United States. Journal of Religion and Health. 2022;**62**(3):1810-1831. DOI: 10.1007/s10943-022-01708-0

[38] Dyer NL, Baldwin AL, Rand WL. A large-scale effectiveness trial of Reiki for physical and psychological health. The Journal of Alternative and Complementary Medicine. 2019;**25**(12):1156-1162. DOI: 10.1089/acm.2019.0022

[39] Bagci H, Yucel SC. A systematic review of the studies about therapeutic touch after the year of 2000. International Journal of Caring Sciences. 2020;**13**(1):231-241. Available from: https://www.internationaljournalofcaringsciences.org/docs/27_bassi_original_13_1.pdf

[40] Sinatra ST, Sinatra DS, Sinatra SW, Chevalier G. Grounding - the universal anti-inflammatory remedy. Biomedical Journal. 2023;**46**(Special Edition):11-16

[41] Soliman J, Elsanadi R, Messele F, Kelly KM. The effect of combined red, blue, and near-infrared light - emitting diode (LED) photobiomodulation therapy on speed of wound healing after superficial ablative fractional resurfacing. Laser in Medical Science. 2024;**39**:94. DOI: 10.1007/s10103-024-04042-x

[42] Tsai S-R, Hamblin M. Biological effects and medical applications of infrared radiation. Journal of Photochemistry and Photobiology. B. 2017;**170**:197-207. DOI: 10.1016/j.jphotobiol.2017.04.014

[43] Zhang X, Ma Y. Global trends in research on extracorporeal shock wave therapy (ESWT) from 2000 to 2001. BMC Musculoskeletal Disorders. 2023;**24**:312. DOI: 10.1186/s12891-023-06407-9

[44] ItsHaky B. Unschuld, Huang Di Nei Jing Ling Shu. The ancient classic on needle therapy the complete Chinese text with an annotated English translation. Alternative Complementary & Integrative Medicine. 2016;**3**(1):147

[45] Deng T. Practical Diagnosis in Traditional Chinese Medicine. Great Britain: Elsevier; 2004, (Ergil M, Ergil K, Trans.)

[46] Best-Selling Book. 2024. Available from: Guinness World Records.com; https://www.guinnessworldrecords.com/world-records/best-selling-book-of-non-fiction

[47] Johnson L. The Foolishness of the Message Preached an Original Collection of Soul Food Filled Sermons Vol 1. Diamond Bar: Crystal Fountian Publications; 1999

[48] Balboni M, Balboni T. Do Spirituality and Medicine Go Together? USA: Havard Medical School Center for Bioethics; 2019. Available from: https://bioethics.hms.harvard.edu/journal/spirituality-medicine

[49] Swihart DL, Yarrarapu SN, Martin RL. Cultrural Religious Competence in Clinical Practice. Treasure Island (FL): StatPearls Publishing; 2023, Available from: https://www.ncbi.nlm.nih.gov/books/NBK493216/

[50] Koenig HG. Spirituality in Patient Care: Why, How, When, and What. 3rd ed. West Conshohocken: Templeton Press; 2002

[51] Koenig HG. Spirituality in Patient Care: Why, How, When, and What. 3rd ed. West Conshohocken: Templeton Press; 2007

[52] Koenig HG. Spirituality in Patient Care: Why, How, When, and What. 3rd ed. West Conshohocken: Templeton Press; 2013

[53] Paloutzian RF, Park CL. Handbook of the Psychology of Religion and Spirituality. New York: The Guilford Press; 2005

[54] Mueller PS, Plevak DJ, Rummans TA. Religion, spirituality, and medicine. Mayo Clinic Proceedings. 2001;**76**:1225-1235

[55] Koenig HG. Spiritual aspects of surgery. Ophthalmology Clinics of North America. 2000;**13**(1):71-84

[56] Mavros MN, Athanasiou S, Gkegkes ID, Polyzos KA, Pappas G, Falagas ME. Do psychological variables affect surgical recovery? PLoS One. 2011;**6**(5):1-5

[57] Barsotti TJ, Jain S, Guarneri M, King RP, Vicario D, Mills PJ. An exploratory investigation of human biofield responses to encountering a sacred object. Explore. 2023;**5**:689-694. DOI: 10.1016/j.explore.2023.01.007

[58] Koenig HG. Religion, spirituality, and health: A review and update. Advances in Mind-Body Medicine. 2015;**29**(3):19-26

[59] World Health Organization (WHO). Constitution. 2021. Available from: https://www.who.int/about/governance/constitution

[60] Aluyi-Osa G, Mutali MJ, Zeppieri M. Jackson Cross Cylinder. Treasure Island, FL, USA: StatPearls Publishing; 2023, Bookshelf ID: NBK587353. Available from: https://pubmed.ncbi.nlm.nih.gov/36508527/

[61] Harris WF. The Jackson cross-cylinder. Part 1: Properties. African Vision and Eye Health. 2007;**22**(2):41-55. DOI: 10.4102/aveh.v66i2.218

[62] Sajja A, Puchalski C. Medicine and society training physicians as healers. AMA Journal of Ethics. 2018;**20**(7):655-663

[63] Puchalski CM. The role of spirituality in health care. In: Charlotte Johnson Barrett Lectureship University Medical Center Baylor University Medical Center (BUMC Proceedings 14). Washington DC: The George Washington Institue for Spirituality and Health (GWish) George Washington University; 2001. pp. 352-357

[64] Emoto M. The Hidden Messages in Water. Korea: Atria Books a trademark of Simon & Schuster, Inc; 2001

Chapter 2

Exploring New Frontiers in Alternative Medicine: Insights and Perspectives

Veeresh Pratap and Durga Prasad Beda

Abstract

This paper examines the rise of alternative medicine, explores its new frontiers, and provides important insights and perspectives. Alternative medicine has become an important complement to traditional medical practices due to the increasing number of people seeking a holistic approach to health, and it is natural this research examines various alternative therapies, such as acupuncture, herbs, chiropractic care, and homeopathy, and tests their effectiveness, safety, and integration into and management of primary health care, e.g., legal issues, scientific evidence, and ability to integrate with traditional medicine. Through a comprehensive review of recent research, expert opinion, and case studies, this paper aims to provide nuanced understandings of the potential and limitations of alternative medicine and highlight its role in the health of the future of the emphasis. The insights gleaned from this study may provide valuable perspectives for health care providers, researchers, and patients considering alternative therapies.

Keywords: alternative medicine, herbal medicine, chiropractic care, homeopathy, acupuncture, holistic approach

1. Introduction

1.1 Definition and scope

1.1.1 Definition

Alternative medicine refers to a range of medical therapies and practices that are not typically part of conventional (mainstream) medicine. It includes a variety of approaches that are used instead of traditional treatments. The phrase refers to a wide range of methods, principles, and techniques that require the use of natural or holistic approaches to promote well-being and healing [1].

1.1.2 Scope

The practice of alternative medicine is broad and encompasses a wide range of practices and therapies outside the scope of traditional western medicine.

These include herbal medicine, acupuncture, homeopathy, chiropractic, naturopathy, and more. Alternative medicine tends to focus on holistic approaches, emphasizing the body's ability to heal itself and the integration of mind, body, and spirit [2]. It is often used in conjunction with traditional healing, especially in the management of chronic conditions, pain, and stress. While some new treatments have been scientifically validated, others remain controversial and may vary in effectiveness. The popularity of alternative medicine has gained momentum worldwide, with patients interested in natural cures, preventive care, and personalized healthcare [3–5].

1.2 Overview of major alternative medicine practices

Alternative medicine incorporates modalities beyond traditional western medicine. Below is a brief summary of some common reactions in alternative formulations:

1. *Acupuncture*

    - *Origin*: Traditional Chinese Medicine (TCM).
    - *Principle*: Thin needles are inserted into specific areas of the body to balance the flow of energy (Qi).
    - *Uses*: Pain management, stress reduction, and treatment of various conditions like migraines, arthritis, and insomnia [6].

2. *Ayurveda*

    - *Origin*: Ancient India.
    - *Principle*: It focuses on balancing the three evils (Vata, Pitta, and Kapha) through diet, lifestyle, and herbs.
    - *Uses*: Holistic health, detoxification, and treating chronic diseases [7].

3. *Homeopathy*

    - *Origin*: Germany, developed by Samuel Hahnemann in the eighteenth century.
    - *Principle*: Based on the principle of "like cures like," the use of highly concentrated ingredients to stimulate the body's natural healing response.
    - *Uses*: Treating allergies, asthma, depression, and skin conditions [8].

4. *Naturopathy*

    - *Origin*: Developed in Europe and North America in the nineteenth century.
    - *Principle*: It emphasizes natural healing with a variety of therapies, including nutrition, herbal medicine, and physical therapy.
    - *Uses*: Preventive care, chronic disease management, and overall wellness [9].

5. *Chiropractic*

- *Origin*: United States, developed by Daniel David Palmer in the nineteenth century.
- *Principle*: It focuses on the diagnosis and treatment of mechanical dysfunction of the musculoskeletal system, especially the spine.
- *Uses*: Back pain, neck pain, and improving overall musculoskeletal health [10].

6. *Herbal medicine*

- *Origin*: Various cultures worldwide, including TCM, Ayurveda, and western herbalism.
- *Principle*: It uses plant-based products because of their chemical properties.
- *Uses:* Treating a wide range of conditions from digestive issues to skin disorders [11].

7. *Reiki*

- *Origin*: Japan, developed by Mikao Usui in the early twentieth century.
- *Principle*: An energy healing technique in which healers use their hands to transfer energy to the patient to promote healing.
- *Uses*: Stress reduction, relaxation, and enhancing overall well-being [12].

8. *Traditional Chinese Medicine (TCM)*

- *Origin*: Ancient China.
- *Principle*: A holistic approach including acupuncture, herbs, cupping, and tai chi, focused on balancing yin and yang.
- *Uses*: Treating a variety of conditions, including digestive issues, respiratory problems, and stress [13].

9. *Osteopathy*

- *Origin*: United States, developed by Andrew Taylor Still in the nineteenth century.
- *Principle*: It emphasizes the relationship between the structure and function of the body and the body's ability to heal.
- *Uses*: Musculoskeletal pain, improving circulation, and enhancing overall health [14].

10. *Aromatherapy*

- *Origin*: Ancient civilizations, including Egypt and India.
- *Principle*: Uses essential oils from plants for therapeutic purposes.
- *Uses:* Stress relief, mood enhancement, and alleviating symptoms of various conditions like headaches and insomnia [15].

11. *Meditation and mindfulness*

- *Origin:* Ancient practices with roots in Buddhism and Hinduism.
- *Principle*: Focus on the mind-body connection to promote mental clarity, relaxation, and emotional well-being.
- *Uses*: Stress reduction, anxiety, depression, and enhancing overall quality of life [16].

12. *Yoga*

- *Origin*: Ancient India.
- *Principle*: It combines physical posture, breath control, meditation, and ethical practices for overall well-being.
- *Uses*: Physical fitness, stress management, and improving mental health [17].

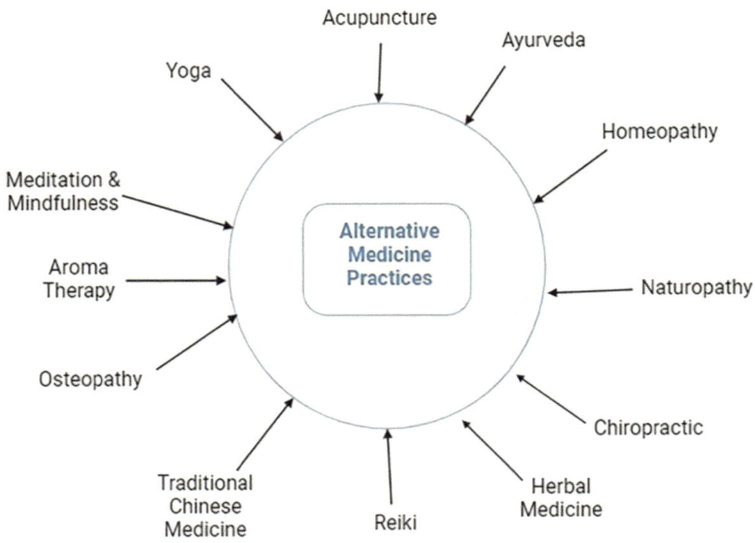

Figure 1.
Schematic diagram of various practices of alternative medicine.

Each of these practices has a unique approach to health and healing, and many people combine them with traditional healing to achieve optimal health and wellness (**Figure 1**).

2. Traditional Chinese Medicine (TCM)

Qi (life force), the five elements, and yin and yang are the pillars of Traditional Chinese Medicine (TCM) thought. They symbolize yin and yang, the harmony of opposite but complementary energies in the body and the universe. The five elements—wood, fire, earth, metal, and water—are supposed to control various physiological processes and pathological changes in the body and are considered essential elements of life as they pass through the qi meridians. Qi must be balanced and flow properly for good health; dysfunction can lead to illness. TCM uses diagnostic techniques such as tongue tests, pulse readings, and observations to regulate the balance of yin, yang, and qi. Acupuncture, herbal medicine, food therapy, and Qi-Gong exercises are some of the treatments that attempt to restore harmony. To achieve health and well-being, TCM generally emphasizes a holistic approach that sees the body as an integrated whole and takes into account the relationships between environmental, emotional, and physiological components [18–21].

2.1 Acupuncture and moxibustion

Acupuncture and moxibustion are integral parts of Traditional Chinese Medicine (TCM), which is widely recognized as innovative medical practices. Acupuncture involves inserting microneedles into specific areas on the body to stimulate the body's energy flow, or "Qi," called acupoints [22]. This practice is believed to restore balance and enhance natural healing by channeling meridians they are targeted, which are the internal pathways of Qi. In some areas, the dried plant moxa (usually mugwort) is burned near or on the skin. The heat from moxibustion is thought to raise the qi, improve blood circulation, and nourish the strength of the immune system [23–25]. Together, acupuncture and moxibustion are used to treat a wide range of conditions, including chronic pain, digestive issues, and stress-related problems, providing a holistic approach to health and well-being [26–28].

2.2 Herbal medicine

Plants or plant extracts used for medicinal purposes are herbal remedies commonly referred to as herbal remedies or plant remedies. It is one of the oldest forms of medicine in the world and has been used in many different cultures. Here is a summary of some important facts about herbs:

2.2.1 Principles

- *Holistic approach*: Herbs generally take a holistic approach, considering the whole person (body, mind, and spirit) rather than just treating symptoms.
- *Natural remedies*: Plants have chemical compounds from their leaves, stems, flowers, seeds, and leaf parts.

- *Balance and harmony*: Many traditions, such as TCM and Ayurveda, emphasize balancing and harmonizing the body's energies within the body and the environment [29].

2.2.2 Common herbs and their uses

- *Echinacea*: Often used to boost the immune system and fight colds.
- *St. John's Wort*: Commonly used for mild to moderate depression.
- *Ginger*: Known for its anti-nausea and digestive properties.
- *Turmeric*: Used for its anti-inflammatory and antioxidant effects.
- *Ginseng*: Believed to boost energy, reduce stress, and improve cognitive function [30].

3. Ayurveda

3.1 Origins and philosophy

Ayurveda is a comprehensive system of medicine that dates back more than 5000 years and originated in ancient India. Combining the Sanskrit words "ayur" (life) and "veda" (knowledge), its name is taken from this language, indicating its strength in terms of life and health. The concept of a wonderful balance of mental, physical, and spiritual well-being is central to Ayurvedic philosophy [31–33]. Many factors, including nutrition, herbs, exercise, meditation, and lifestyle decisions, all influence this balance. According to Ayurveda, human beings are divided into three distinct mind-body types called Doshas (Vata, Pitta, and Kapha), each with specific

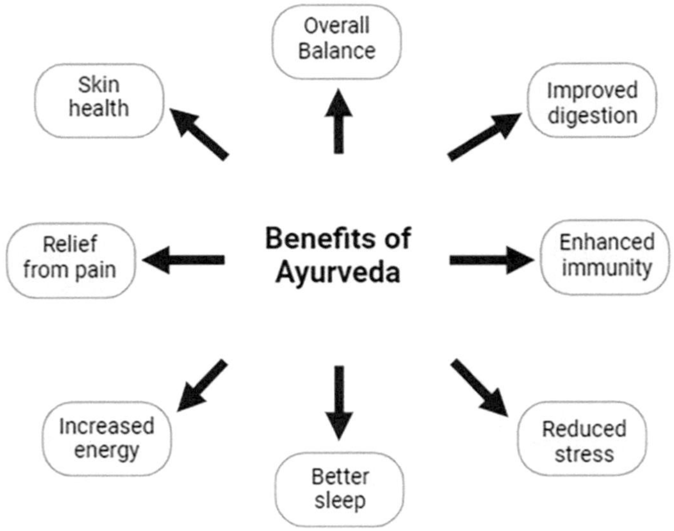

Figure 2.
Schematic diagram of benefits of Ayurveda system of medicine.

DOI: http://dx.doi.org/10.5772/intechopen.1007402

physical and mental characteristics. The main goal of Ayurvedic practices through individual and natural methods is to harmonize these evils to avoid diseases and achieve optimal health [34–36].

3.2 Doshas and their significance

Doshas are fundamental concepts in Ayurveda, the traditional Indian system of medicine. They represent the three most important energies or principles that govern physical and mental processes in the body—Vata, Pitta, and Kapha [37]. Gases made of air and ether are associated with movement and creation; gall, made of fire and water, regulates food, metabolism, and transformation, while wetlands with soil and water are associated with structure, stability, and resistance to disease. These evils are balanced or unbalanced and determine a person's health, temperament, and propensity to certain diseases [38]. Ayurvedic medicine focuses on restoring the balance between the Doshas through diet, lifestyle changes, herbs, and other practices aimed at promoting overall well-being and preventing disease. Understanding the basic dosha can help for individual treatments to integrate physically and mentally (**Figure 2**) [39, 40].

4. Homeopathy

4.1 Foundational principles

Samuel Hahnemann established a new system of homeopathy in the 1700s. Two basic ideas form its foundation: the law of equality and the law of infinity. Generally, according to a similar rule summarized as "like cures like," a drug that causes symptoms in healthy individuals can be used to treat the same symptom in a patient. The idea behind this phenomenon is that as water is added, the strength of a substance increases. In addition, homeopathy emphasizes personalized care, in which prescriptions are based on the specific symptoms and overall health of the patient. This holistic approach considers a person's emotional and mental health in addition to their physical symptoms [39, 41–43].

4.2 Preparation and potency of remedies

Homeopathic remedies are manufactured through a process called potentization, which involves slow dilution and infusion (vigorous shaking). The process starts with a base, which can be plant minerals or animal products, and is then mixed with alcohol or water. This mixture is vigorously shaken in a process called inheritance, which is believed to enhance the medicine's healing properties [44]. The dilution process is repeated several times, with each successive dilution increasing the potency of the remedy homeopathically, though decreasing the availability of the original. The final product is considered strong in homeopathy even though it has been synthesized greater; though, it is believed to stimulate the body's natural healing response. The number indicates the number of steps for attenuation, and the letters represent the attenuation ratio [45].

4.3 Common homeopathic treatments

Homeopathic remedies are widely used for a variety of health conditions, with remedies often based on a person's symptoms and overall code. Some common homeopathic remedies are *Arnica montana*, which is commonly used for wounds, ulcers, and muscle pain; Nux vomica, often recommended for digestive issues, including constipation, indigestion, and constipation, especially those associated with stress or overeating; and Ignatia amara, often used for emotional distress, especially grief or anxiety [46–48]. Another popular treatment is oscillococcine, which is often used to relieve flu symptoms. Homeopaths also frequently prescribe belladonna for high fevers and inflammation and *Rhus toxicodendron* for joint pain and stiffness, especially when symptoms improve with movement. These treatments are based on a "like treatment like" principle, where the causes of symptoms in a healthy person are very diluted. The patient is treated for the same symptoms [49–52].

5. Naturopathy

5.1 Core principles of naturopathic medicine

Naturopathic medicine is based on several core principles that guide its practice. These principles focus on holistic, preventive, and natural approaches to healthcare. Here are the core principles:

1. *The healing power of nature (vis medicatrix naturae)*: Naturopathic medicine recognizes the body's inherent ability to heal itself. Naturopathic doctors (NDs) work to support and enhance this natural healing process.

2. *Identify and treat the causes (tolle causam)*: Naturopathic physicians aim to identify and address the root causes of illness rather than merely treating symptoms. By finding and treating the underlying cause, long-term healing and health can be achieved.

3. *First, do no harm (primum non nocere)*: Naturopathic doctors adhere to treatments and interventions that are safe and effective, minimizing the risk of harmful side effects. They use the simplest techniques necessary for diagnosis and care.

4. *Doctor as teacher (docere)*: One of the most important aspects of natural medicine is educating patients about their well-being. NDs provide patients with the information and resources they need to manage their health.

5. *Treat the whole person*: An individual's physical, emotional, psychological, genetic, environmental, social, and spiritual well-being are all considered through a holistic approach to natural disease. Individualized treatment plans are developed to treat each patient, addressing specific needs.

6. *Prevention*: The focus is on using natural therapies and healthy lifestyle choices to promote wellness and prevent disease. NDs collaborate with patients to better identify risk factors and establish preventive measures [53–55].

These concepts form the cornerstone of biomedicine and guide biomedical practitioners toward a comprehensive patient-centered approach to promoting optimal health and well-being.

5.2 Naturopathic treatments (hydrotherapy, nutrition, etc.)

Naturopathic medicine, which includes practices such as hydrotherapy and nutritional therapy, represents a holistic approach to medicine, emphasizing the body's natural ability to heal itself. Hydrotherapy uses water in a variety of ways—such as baths, hot water, and compression—as therapeutic stimulants for circulation, detoxification, and overall well-being. Nutrition focuses on the use of food and natural supplements to prevent and treat the body's physiological processes [56]. These therapies are often combined with comprehensive biological programs that include other natural therapies, such as combining herbal medicine, acupuncture, and lifestyle counseling for long-term health by enhancing natural defenses. This approach, which is also being enhanced, appeals to those seeking natural, preventive, patient-centered care of the greater [57–59].

6. Herbal medicine

6.1 History and development of herbal practices

Herbal medicine is old and dates back to ancient civilizations when early humans relied on plants for healing. Many ancient Greek, Chinese, Indian, and Egyptian cultures have recorded plants used in their texts in Ayurveda, Ebers, Papyrus, etc. Hippocrates and Dioscorides made significant contributions to medicine in ancient Greece; the "De Materia Medica" of Dioscorides became the dominant herbal knowledge for many years. Comprehensive data on hundreds of plants are provided by the Chinese Materia Medica, compiled during the Han Dynasty [60]. In the Middle Ages, herbal methods were preserved and developed by monastic institutions in Europe; in the Islamic world, for example, scientists such as Avicenna combined Persian, Greek, and Roman knowledge. The printing press and the Age of Discovery, which brought new plants from the Americas and other continents, led to a rebirth of medicinal plant study and cataloging throughout the Renaissance period and an increase in contact with cultural traditions [61].

6.2 Safety, efficacy, and regulatory issues

Herbal medicines based on plants and plant extracts are fraught with safety, efficacy, and regulatory challenges. Major safety issues and potential side effects and prescription drug additives. Side effects of herbal remedies can range from minor gastrointestinal problems to severe diarrhea or liver toxicity in sensitive people, suggesting that natural products do not prove safe either, because they vary between batches and brands. Strength and purity can vary widely, as well as changes in product characteristics and standards of performance that pose additional risks [62].

Evaluating the effectiveness of herbs is another daunting obstacle. Compared to pharmaceuticals, the scientific evidence for their efficacy is much more limited, due to the lack of well-designed clinical trials and differentiated study methodologies.

Further complicating matters is the wide variation in regulation between countries when it comes to herbal medicines. Because these products are classified more as dietary supplements than drugs, there are few stringent regulations governing safety and efficacy testing before they are allowed for sale. This regulatory approach can have resulted in inconsistent or similar safety and product quality requirements.

Increased research funding to test efficacy, harmonization of regulatory frameworks in a global marketplace, and quality control standards are all important elements of a robust approach to challenges in this. Herbal medicines have the potential to overcome these obstacles and provide useful therapies in addition to conventional therapies, as long as safety, efficacy, and regulatory issues are carefully monitored and followed [63, 64].

7. Energy medicine

7.1 Concepts of energy healing

Energy medicine includes a variety of alternative therapeutic modalities that work on the body's energy utilization or balance to promote physical, emotional, and spiritual well-being. The concept is based on the belief that disturbances in the body's energy system or imbalances can manifest as disease. Practitioners of energy healing techniques, such as Reiki, Qi-Gong, or therapeutic touch, use a variety of techniques to channel, manipulate, or balance the flow of energy. Though scientifically recognized as such, these practices tend to be relatively minor. Energy healing techniques that report benefits such as pain relief and improved mood are often included in traditional medicine as complementary medicine to promote health and comprehensive treatment plans [65–67].

7.2 Reiki, Healing Touch, and other modalities

Reiki, Healing Touch, and other similar modalities fall under the category of energy healing practices. These methods aim to promote healing and wellness by manipulating the body's energy fields. Here's a brief overview of each:

7.2.1 Reiki

Reiki is a Japanese technique for stress reduction and relaxation that also promotes healing. It is based on the idea that an unseen "life force energy" flows through us and is what causes us to be alive. If one's life force energy is low, then we are more likely to get sick or feel stress, and if it is high, we are more capable of being happy and healthy. A Reiki practitioner channels this energy through their hands to the patient, usually without physical touch, to encourage emotional or physical healing [68].

7.2.2 Healing Touch

Healing Touch is an energy therapy in which practitioners consciously use their hands in a heart-centered and intentional way to support and facilitate physical, emotional, mental, and spiritual health. Developed by Janet Mentgen in the 1980s, it involves light touch or near-body touch to clear, balance, and energize the human energy system, promoting self-healing [69].

8. Chiropractic and osteopathic medicine

8.1 Principles and techniques

Chiropractic and osteopathic medicine are alternative forms of health care that focus on the diagnosis, treatment, and prevention of musculoskeletal diseases and emphasize the body's own healing powers. Chiropractic is primarily concerned with the use of the spine and other joints, including the musculoskeletal systems, especially the spine, which is believed to be well aligned to allow the body to heal without surgery or drugs. Manual spine manipulation and other therapies are used to restore mobility of joints with muscle injuries due to traumatic events such as falls or common stresses, such as sitting with poor back support [70].

Osteopathic medicine, while having some similarities to osteopathy, is broader in scope. Osteopaths (DOs) are fully licensed physicians who practice in all areas of medicine but also have specialized training in musculoskeletal systems. They use a holistic, conscious approach to medicine that emphasizes the relationship between structure and function. Orthopedic techniques include osteopathic manipulation (OMT), in which physicians manually diagnose, treat, and prevent disease or injury. OMT can involve stretching, gentle compression, and resistance to promote healing. The underlying principle of osteoporosis is that the body has an innate ability to heal itself, and OMT is used to enhance this natural process [71].

Both osteopathic medicine and osteopathic medicine emphasize a controlled approach to alcohol use, but osteopathic medicine incorporates a wide range of therapies and is added to traditional medicine, while osteopathic therapy focuses more on the use of the spine and joints [8, 72–76].

9. Conclusion

Incorporating a wide range of practices, including alternative medicine, herbal medicine, acupuncture, chiropractic, homeopathy, etc. It has attracted a great deal of attention and has been used worldwide. Its appeal lies largely in its holistic approach, emphasizing healing of the whole person—mind, body, and spirit—rather than just disease symptoms, which are turned to alternative therapies to seek a less invasive alternative or when conventional treatment fails to provide relief. This approach can give a person a greater sense of commitment to their health and wellness journey.

However, the efficacy and safety of alternative agents remain a matter of ongoing debate. While some interventions have shown benefit and have been incorporated into mainstream health care, others lack strong scientific evidence. Potential interactions between new treatments and conventional medications also raise concerns. It is important for patients to consult with healthcare professionals before starting any new treatment to ensure it is compatible with their overall treatment plan. As the medical profession continues to evolve, incorporating new evidence-based practices into traditional health care delivery can enhance patient outcomes and improve access to care, which can be selected.

Acknowledgements

I would like to extend my deepest gratitude to the following individuals and institutions for their invaluable support and contributions to this chapter:

First and foremost, I am profoundly grateful to Dr. J. Rajasekhar for his guidance, encouragement, and insightful feedback throughout the writing process. Their expertise and support were instrumental in shaping this work.

I would also like to thank Gokaraju Rangaraju College of Pharmacy for providing the necessary resources and a conducive environment for writing. Special thanks to the staff of the Department of Pharmacology for their assistance and collaboration.

A heartfelt thanks to my colleagues and friends, whose discussions and suggestions greatly enriched this chapter. Your intellectual and moral support kept me motivated and focused.

Finally, I owe a special debt of gratitude to my family for their unwavering support and understanding during this endeavor. Your love and patience have been my greatest source of strength.

Authors acknowledge the use of ChatGPT for language polishing of the manuscript.

Thank you all for making this work possible.

Conflict of interest

The authors declare no conflict of interest.

Author details

Veeresh Pratap[1*] and Durga Prasad Beda[2]

1 Gokaraju Rangaraju College of Pharmacy, Hyderabad, Telangana, India

2 GITAM School of Pharmacy, Hyderabad, Telangana, India

*Address all correspondence to: pratap.veeresh@gmail.com

References

[1] The Impact of Alternative Medicine in the 21st Century. Available from: https://sourceessay.com/the-impact-of-alternative-medicine-in-the-21st-century/

[2] Cyranoski D. China is promoting coronavirus treatments based on unproven traditional medicines. Nature. 2020. DOI: 10.1038/d41586-020-01284-x

[3] Sayligil O. Ethical evaluation of clinical research on complementary and alternative medicine. In: Evidence-Based Medicine. London, UK: IntechOpen; 2020

[4] Alternative Medicine. Disease Prevention and Healthy Lifestyles. Available from: https://courses.lumenlearning.com/diseaseprevention/chapter/alternative-medical-practices/

[5] Hao GA, Xin-Sheng YA. Strengthen the research on the medicinal and edible substances to advance the development of the comprehensive healthcare industry of TCMs. Chinese Journal of Natural Medicines. 2019;**17**(1):1-2. DOI: 10.1016/S1875-5364(19)30002-0

[6] Srinivasan R, Sugumar VR. Spread of traditional medicines in India: Results of national sample survey organization's perception survey on use of Ayush. Journal of Evidence-Based Complementary & Alternative Medicine. 2017;**22**(2):194-204. DOI: 10.1177/2156587215607673

[7] Kumnerdkhonkaen P, Saenglee S, Asgar MA, Senawong G, Khongsukwiwat K, Senawong T. Antiproliferative activities and phenolic acid content of water and ethanolic extracts of the powdered formula of *Houttuynia cordata* Thunb. fermented broth and *Phyllanthus emblica* Linn. fruit. BMC Complementary and Alternative Medicine. 2018;**18**(1):130. DOI: 10.1186/s12906-018-2185-x

[8] Payyappallimana U, Patwardhan K, Mangalath P, Kessler CS, Jayasundar R, Kizhakkeveettil A, et al. The COVID-19 pandemic and the relevance of ayurveda's whole systems approach to health and disease management. The Journal of Alternative and Complementary Medicine. 2020;**26**(12):1089-1092. DOI: 10.1089/acm.2020.0370

[9] Dong FH. Precise application of Traditional Chinese Medicine in minimally-invasive techniques. Zhongguo Gu Shang = China Journal of Orthopaedics and Traumatology. 2018;**31**(6):493-496. DOI: 10.3969/j.issn.1003-0034.2018.06.001

[10] Ma Y, Chen M, Guo Y, Liu J, Chen W, Guan M, et al. Prevention and treatment of infectious diseases by traditional Chinese medicine: A commentary. APMIS. 2019;**127**:372-384. DOI: 10.1111/apm.12928

[11] Deng G. Integrative medicine therapies for pain management in cancer patients. The Cancer Journal. 2019;**25**(5):343. DOI: 10.1097/PPO.0000000000000399

[12] Jackson C. Trends in the use of complementary health approaches among adults in the United States: New data. Holistic Nursing Practice. 2015;**29**(3):178-179. DOI: 10.1097/HNP.0000000000000088

[13] Rao A, Hickman LD, Sibbritt D, Newton PJ, Phillips JL. Is energy healing an effective non-pharmacological

therapy for improving symptom management of chronic illnesses? A systematic review. Complementary Therapies in Clinical Practice. 2016;**25**:26-41. DOI: 10.1016/j.ctcp.2016.07.003

[14] Yeung A, Chan JS, Cheung JC, Zou L. Qigong and Tai-Chi for mood regulation. Focus. 2018;**16**(1):40-47. DOI: 10.1176/appi.focus.20170042

[15] Grossman LD, Roscoe R, Shack AR. Complementary and alternative medicine for diabetes. Canadian Journal of Diabetes. 2018;**42**:S154-S161. DOI: 10.1016/j.jcjd.2017.10.023

[16] Buckner CA, Lafrenie RM, Dénommée JA, Caswell JM, Want DA. Complementary and alternative medicine use in patients before and after a cancer diagnosis. Current Oncology. 2018;**25**(4):e275. DOI: 10.3747/co.25.3884

[17] Johnson A, Roberts L, Elkins G. Complementary and alternative medicine for menopause. Journal of Evidence-Based Integrative Medicine. 2019;**24**:2515690X19829380. DOI: 10.1177/2515690X19829380

[18] Burton MS. Complementary and alternative medicine in rehabilitation. Current Sports Medicine Reports. 2019;**18**(8):283-284. DOI: 10.1249/JSR.0000000000000617

[19] WHO. Diabetes. Available from: https://www.who.int/news-room/fact-sheets/detail/diabetes [Accessed: July 23, 2024]

[20] Pang GM, Li FX, Yan Y, Zhang Y, Kong LL, Zhu P, et al. Herbal medicine in the treatment of patients with type 2 diabetes mellitus. Chinese Medical Journal. 2019;**132**(1):78. DOI: 10.1097/CM9.0000000000000006

[21] Tian J, Jin D, Bao Q, Ding Q, Zhang H, Gao Z, et al. Evidence and potential mechanisms of traditional Chinese medicine for the treatment of type 2 diabetes: A systematic review and meta-analysis. Diabetes, Obesity and Metabolism. 2019;**21**(8):1801-1816. DOI: 10.1111/dom.13760

[22] Necyk C, Zubach-Cassano L. Natural health products and diabetes: A practical review. Canadian Journal of Diabetes. 2017;**41**(6):642-647. DOI: 10.1016/j.jcjd.2017.06.014

[23] Chen L, Deng H, Cui H, Fang J, Zuo Z, Deng J, et al. Inflammatory responses and inflammation-associated diseases in organs. Oncotarget. 2018;**9**(6):7204. DOI: 10.18632/oncotarget.23208

[24] Bower JE, Irwin MR. Mind–body therapies and control of inflammatory biology: A descriptive review. Brain, Behavior, and Immunity. 2016;**51**:1-1. DOI: 10.1016/j.bbi.2015.06.012

[25] Lawal IO, Olufade II, Rafiu BO, Aremu AO. Ethnobotanical survey of plants used for treating cough associated with respiratory conditions in Ede South local government area of Osun State, Nigeria. Plants. 2020;**9**(5):647. DOI: 10.3390/plants9050647

[26] Lee JH, Min DS, Lee CW, Song KH, Kim YS, Kim HP. Ginsenosides from Korean Red Ginseng ameliorate lung inflammatory responses: Inhibition of the MAPKs/NF-κB/c-Fos pathways. Journal of Ginseng Research. 2018;**42**(4):476-484. DOI: 10.1016/j.jgr.2017.05.005

[27] Younis W, Asif H, Sharif A, Riaz H, Bukhari IA, Assiri AM. Traditional medicinal plants used for respiratory disorders in Pakistan: A review of the ethno-medicinal and pharmacological

evidence. Chinese Medicine. 2018;**13**(1):1-29. DOI: 10.1186/s13020-018-0204-y

[28] Kohn CM, Paudyal P. A systematic review and meta-analysis of complementary and alternative medicine in asthma. European Respiratory Review. 2017;**26**(143):160092. DOI: 10.1183/16000617.0092-2016

[29] Radiation Therapy Side Effects. Available from: https://www.cancer.org/treatment/treatments-and-side-effects/treatment-types/radiation/effects-on-different-parts-of-body.html [Accessed: July 23, 2024]

[30] Luo Q, Asher GN. Complementary and alternative medicine use at a comprehensive cancer center. Integrative Cancer Therapy. 2017;**16**(1):104-109. DOI: 10.1177/1534735416643384

[31] Knecht K, Kinder D, Stockert A. Biologically-based complementary and alternative medicine (CAM) use in cancer patients: The good, the bad, the misunderstood. Frontiers in Nutrition. 2020;**6**:196. DOI: 10.3389/fnut.2019.00196

[32] Kievisiene J, Jautakyte R, Rauckiene-Michaelsson A, Fatkulina N, Agostinis-Sobrinho C. The effect of art therapy and music therapy on breast cancer patients: What we know and what we need to find out—A systematic review. Evidence-Based Complementary and Alternative Medicine. 2020;**2020**:1-14. DOI: 10.1155/2020/7390321

[33] Bray F, Ferlay J, Soerjomataram I, Siegel RL, Torre LA, Jemal A. Global cancer statistics 2018: GLOBOCAN estimates of incidence and mortality worldwide for 36 cancers in 185 countries. CA: A Cancer Journal for Clinicians. 2018;**68**(6):394-424. DOI: 10.3322/caac.21492

[34] Zaid H, Silbermann M, Amash A, Gincel D, Abdel-Sattar E, Sarikahya NB. Medicinal plants and natural active compounds for cancer chemoprevention/chemotherapy. Evidence-Based Complementary and Alternative Medicine. 2017;**2017**:7952417. DOI: 10.1155/2017/7952417

[35] Greenlee H, DuPont-Reyes MJ, Balneaves LG, Carlson LE, Cohen MR, Deng G, et al. Clinical practice guidelines on the evidence-based use of integrative therapies during and after breast cancer treatment. CA: A Cancer Journal for Clinicians. 2017;**67**(3):194-232. DOI: 10.3322/caac.21397

[36] Alternative Cancer Treatments: 10 Options to Consider. Available from: https://www.mayoclinic.org/diseases-conditions/cancer/in-depth/cancer-treatment/art-20047246 [Accessed: July 23, 2024]

[37] Coakley AB, Barron AM. Energy therapies in oncology nursing. Seminars in Oncology Nursing. 2012;**28**(1):55-63

[38] Habli Z, Toumieh G, Fatfat M, Rahal ON, Gali-Muhtasib H. Emerging cytotoxic alkaloids in the battle against Cancer: Overview of molecular mechanisms. Molecules. 2017;**22**(2):250. DOI: 10.3390/molecules22020250

[39] Shaito A, Thuan DTB, Phu HT, Nguyen THD, Hasan H, Halabi S, et al. Herbal medicine for cardiovascular diseases: Efficacy, mechanisms, and safety. Frontiers in Pharmacology. 7 Apr 2020;**11**:422. DOI: 10.3389/fphar.2020.00422

[40] Bronzato S, Durante A. Dietary supplements and cardiovascular diseases. International Journal of Preventive Medicine. 2018;**9**:1-8. DOI: 10.4103/ijpvm.IJPVM_179_17

[41] de Lima PR, Duque AP, Moreira BR, Junior LF. Acupuncture for the treatment of cardiovascular diseases: A systematic review. Journal of Acupuncture and Meridian Studies. 2019;**12**(2):43-51. DOI: 10.1016/j.jams.2018.07.005

[42] Rastogi S, Pandey MM, Rawat AK. Traditional herbs: A remedy for cardiovascular disorders. Phytomedicine. 2016;**23**(11):1082-1089. DOI: 10.1016/j.phymed.2015.10.012

[43] Sun YE, Wang W, Qin J. Anti-hyperlipidemia of garlic by reducing the level of total cholesterol and low-density lipoprotein: A meta-analysis. Medicine. 2018;**97**(18):e0255. DOI: 10.1097/MD.0000000000010255

[44] Alternative Treatments for Insomnia. Available from: https://www.webmd.com/sleep-disorders/alternative-treatments-for-insomnia [Accessed: July 23, 2024]

[45] Tordjman S, Chokron S, Delorme R, Charrier A, Bellissant E, Jaafari N, et al. Melatonin: Pharmacology, functions and therapeutic benefits. Current Neuropharmacology. 2017;**15**(3):434-443. DOI: 10.2174/1570159X14666161228122115

[46] Velasco-Rodríguez R, Pérez-Hernández MG, Maturano-Melgoza JA, Hilerio-López ÁG, Monroy-Rojas A, Arana-Gómez B, et al. The effect of aromatherapy with lavender (*Lavandula angustifolia*) on serum melatonin levels. Complementary Therapies in Medicine. 2019;**47**:102208. DOI: 10.1016/j.ctim.2019.102208

[47] Hmwe NT, Browne G, Mollart L, Allanson V, Chan SW. Acupressure to improve sleep quality of older people in residential aged care: A randomised controlled trial protocol. Trials. 2020;**21**:360. DOI: 10.1186/s13063-020-04286-2

[48] Banno M, Harada Y, Taniguchi M, Tobita R, Tsujimoto H, Tsujimoto Y, et al. Exercise can improve sleep quality: A systematic review and meta-analysis. Peer J. 2018;**6**:e5172. DOI: 10.7717/peerj.5172

[49] Pera A. Cognitive, behavioral, and emotional disorders in populations affected by the COVID-19 outbreak. Frontiers in Psychology. 2020;**11**:2263. DOI: 10.3389/fpsyg.2020.02263

[50] Ostuzzi G, Papola D, Gastaldon C, Schoretsanitis G, Bertolini F, Amaddeo F, et al. Safety of psychotropic medications in people with COVID-19: Evidence review and practical recommendations. BMC Medicine. 2020;**18**(1):1-4. DOI: 10.1186/s12916-020-01685-9

[51] Liu K, Chen Y, Wu D, Lin R, Wang Z, Pan L. Effects of progressive muscle relaxation on anxiety and sleep quality in patients with COVID-19. Complementary Therapies in Clinical Practice. 2020;**39**:101132. DOI: 10.1016/j.ctcp.2020.101132

[52] Loewy J. Music therapy as a potential intervention for sleep improvement. Nature and Science of Sleep. 2020;**12**:1. DOI: 10.2147/NSS.S194938

[53] Trahan T, Durrant SJ, Müllensiefen D, Williamson VJ. The music that helps people sleep and the reasons they believe it works: A mixed methods analysis of online survey reports. PLoS ONE. 2018;**13**(11):e0206531. DOI: 10.1371/journal.pone.0206531

[54] Gupta R. Integrating ayurveda with modern medicine for enhanced patient care: Analysis of realities. The Physician. 2024;**9**(1):1-6. DOI: 10.38192/1.9.1.3

[55] Akter S, Nazmul Hasan M, Rokeya B, Akhter H, Shamim Gazi M,

Sabrin F, et al. Alternative Medicine: A Recent Overview. IntechOpen; 2021. DOI: 10.5772/intechopen.97039

[56] Rizvi SAA, Einstein GP, Tulp OL, Sainvil F, Branly R. Introduction to traditional medicine and their role in prevention and treatment of emerging and re-emerging diseases. Biomolecules. 2022;**12**(10):1442. DOI: 10.3390/biom12101442

[57] Krsnik S, Erjavec K. Factors influencing use of medicinal herbs. Journal of Patient Experience. 2024;**11**: 1-8. DOI: 10.1177/23743735241241181

[58] Sinkevich D. Health risks of herbal medicine in the US: Recommendations to improve awareness and advance safety. Master's Projects and Capstones. 2023:1571. Available from: https://repository.usfca.edu/capstone/1571

[59] Han H-Y, Han K-H, Ahn J-H, et al. Subchronic toxicity assessment of phytolacca americana L. (Phytolaccaceae) in F344 rats. Natural Product Communications. 2020;**15**(7):1934578X2094165. DOI: 10.1177/1934578X20941656

[60] Zulkhairi Amin FA, Shafiq Cheng MZ, Sabri S, Ismail N, Chan KW, Mohd Esa N, et al. In vivo toxicity assessment of the probiotic *Bacillus amyloliquefaciens* HTI-19 isolated from stingless bee (*Heterotrigona itama*) honey. Nutrients. 2023;**15**(10):2390. DOI: 10.3390/nu15102390

[61] Ostermaier A, Barth N, Linde K. How German general practitioners justify their provision of complementary and alternative medicine—A qualitative study. BMC Complementary Medicine and Therapies. 2020;**20**:111. DOI: 10.1186/s12906-020-02907-6

[62] Hübner J, Mücke R, Micke O, Keinki C. Complementary medicine in uro-oncology. Der Urologe. Ausg. A. 2021;**60**(7):953-962. DOI: 10.1007/s00120-021-01584-8

[63] Zhang C, Chen G, Tang G, et al. Multi-component Chinese medicine formulas for drug discovery: State of the art and future perspectives. Acta Materia Medica. 2023;**2**(1):106-125. DOI: 10.15212/AMM-2022-0049

[64] Courric E, Brinvilier D, Couderc P, Ponce-Mora A, Méril-Mamert V, Sylvestre M, et al. Medicinal plants and plant-based remedies in Grande-Terre: An ethnopharmacological approach. Plants (Basel). 2023;**12**(3):654. DOI: 10.3390/plants12030654

[65] Lawal IO, Rafiu BO, Ale JE, Majebi OE, Aremu AO. Ethnobotanical survey of local flora used for medicinal purposes among indigenous people in five areas in Lagos State, Nigeria. Plants (Basel). 2022;**11**(5):633. DOI: 10.3390/plants11050633

[66] Liaqat I, Hussain S, Abid H, Ahmad I, Arif S, Anwar ul Haq M, et al. An ethnobotanical survey of medicinal plants used for primary health care from Patan Sher Khan and surrounding areas of district Sudhnoti, Azad Jammu and Kashmir, Pakistan. Journal of Applied Research in Plant Sciences. 2020;**4**(01):518-528. DOI: 10.38211/joarps.2023.04.01.62

[67] Tangkiatkumjai M, Boardman H, Walker DM. Potential factors that influence usage of complementary and alternative medicine worldwide: A systematic review. BMC Complementary Medicine and Therapies. 2020;**20**:363. DOI: 10.1186/s12906-020-03157-2

[68] Jothydev K, Banshi S, Arun S, Gopika K, Sunitha J, Vysakh C, et al. Prevalence of complementary and alternate medicine use among people

with diabetes in Kerala, India. International Journal of Diabetes and Technology. 2023;**2**(3):85-89. DOI: 10.4103/ijdt.ijdt_36_23

[69] Adel Mehraban MS, Mosallanejad A, Mohammadi M, Tabatabaei Malazy O, Larijani B. Navigating ethical dilemmas in complementary and alternative medicine: A narrative review. Journal of Medical Ethics and History of Medicine. 2024;**17**

[70] Böhne LÄ, Wirner C, Schoser B, Schröter C, Baum P. Frequency and satisfaction of conventional and complementary or alternative therapies for neuromuscular disorders. Neurological Research and Practice. 2023;**5**(1):53. DOI: 10.1186/s42466-023-00281-5

[71] Nazli T, Kishore J, Khan SA, Heena RA, Khan AA. Knowledge and practices of Unani medicine among patients attending OPD at a tertiary care hospital in North India. International Journal of Healthcare Education & Medical Informatics. 2020;**7**(1&2):10-15

[72] Pengpid S, Peltzer K. Utilization of complementary and traditional medicine practitioners among middle-aged and older adults in India: Results of a national survey in 2017-2018. BMC Complementary Medicine and Therapies. 2021;**21**:262. DOI: 10.1186/s12906-021-03432-w

[73] Subhawa S, Chewonarin T, Banjerdpongchai R. The effects of *Houttuynia cordata* Thunb and *Piper ribesioides* wall extracts on breast carcinoma cell proliferation, migration, invasion and apoptosis. Molecules. 2020;**25**:1196. DOI: 10.3390/molecules25051196

[74] Tesfamariam S, Tesfai F, Hussien L, et al. Traditional medicine among the community of Gash-Barka region, Eritrea: Attitude, societal dependence, and pattern of use. BMC Complementary Medicine and Therapies. 2021;**21**:68. DOI: 10.1186/s12906-021-03247-9

[75] Grace R, Vaz J, Da Costa J. Traditional medicine use in Timor-Leste. BMC Complementary Medicine and Therapies. 2020;**20**(1):165. DOI: 10.1186/s12906-020-02912-9

[76] Zantaraia T, Gozhenko A, Popovych I. Relationships between electrical conductivity of acupuncture points and adaptation hormones. Quality in Sport. 2024;**21**:53009. DOI: 10.12775/QS.2024.21.53009

Section 2

Natural Therapy

Chapter 3

Forest Therapy, Stress, and Immune System: A Health Triangle Approach

Hendro Prabowo and Awal Prasetyo

Abstract

Forest therapy, a practice that involves guided outdoor healing in natural environments, has shown promising effects on stress reduction and immune system enhancement. This chapter adopts a Health Triangle Approach to explore the interconnected relationship between forest therapy, stress levels, and immune function. By synthesizing evidence from various studies, it is clear that forest therapy not only reduces stress by promoting relaxation and increasing parasympathetic nervous activity but also positively impacts immune function by enhancing natural killer cell activity and regulating inflammatory responses. The Health Triangle Approach provides a comprehensive framework for understanding how forest therapy can contribute to overall health and well-being through its dual effects on stress management and immune system support.

Keywords: forest therapy, stress, immune system, health triangle, inflammatory response, psychophysiological benefit

1. Introduction

Forest therapy is a concept that aims to promote physical and mental health by immersing oneself in nature, particularly in the forests [1–3]. The term "forest therapy" is often used reciprocally with forest bathing *Shinrin-yoku* in Japan, *sēn lín yù* in China, and *sanlimyok* in South Korea [4]. Forest therapy is a mindfulness therapy with a forest location as a place of implementation, carrying out activities that can relieve stress and certain medical complaints, as well as encouraging individuals to expose their senses in a natural environment [3].

The Korea Forest Service (KFS) publicized and recommended that the concept of forest therapy as "human immune strengthening and health-promoting activities that utilize various natural elements, such as aromas and landscapes." Forest therapy aims to gain the health benefits of the forest, which differs from forest bathing as an approach that is enhanced and augmented by guided practice [3, 5]. There were some methods used in forest therapy include [2]: forest walks, forest-viewing, a combination of walking in the forest and looking at forest views, therapy programs involving the five human senses, doing relaxing activities in the forest, and therapy based on traditional medicine. The therapy can be experienced both with a guide and without one. Guided forest therapy involves participating in a guided walk or program led by a trained forest therapy guide, who provides "invitations" to slow down and engage with the natural environment. On the other hand, self-guided forest therapy allows individuals to explore the forest on their own, without a guide [1].

On one side, forests have complex ecosystems and contain natural chemicals that can have beneficial effects on human physiology and psychology. Trees in the forest emit volatile organic compounds, called Phytoncides, which serve to protect themselves from insects, but have a calming effect, improving mood and the immune system. In addition, terpenes, another class of organic compounds that are also secreted by plants in forests, have various health benefits for humans, including anti-inflammatory, analgesic, and antibacterial benefits. For instance, terpenes like beta-caryophyllene can help reduce inflammation and alleviate pain by modulating pathways in the body, making them useful for managing chronic pain conditions. Additionally, compounds such as myrcene have been found to enhance pain relief, while terpenes like thymol exhibit antibacterial effects that can inhibit the growth of harmful bacteria, supporting overall immune health and wound healing. Oxygen radicals, a single negative electron molecule of oxygen, are useful for reducing stress and improving overall human well-being [3, 6]. On the other side, people are drawn to nature, particularly forests, due to biophilic motivations, as supported by scientific research. Biophilia, a term first used by psychoanalyst Fromm, and later Wilson. Fromm describes humanity's innate need establishing a non-destructive relationship with the natural environment by cultivating a sense of love for living creatures. This concept emphasizes the deep connection humans have with nature and the benefits derived from interacting with natural settings [7].

Scientific studies have shown that touch with nature is a fundamental *anthropoids* need, not just a societal preference, and plays a crucial role in promoting health and well-being [8, 9]. A study highlights that humans are inherently responsive to the spaces, shapes, sounds, and patterns of nature, indicating a strong attraction to the natural environment [10]. This responsiveness to nature is deeply rooted in human evolution and has significant implications for mental and physical health.

The interrelationship between mental, physical and social health, as well as interactions between pathogens, hosts, and the environment as prerequisites for disease, are well known as "Health Triangle Approach." The World Health Organization (WHO) formulates the concept of health as a condition of complete physical, mental, and social well-being, not just the absence of disease or weakness. One of human rights is to enjoy the highest standard of health, without distinction of race, religion, political choice, and economic or social status. Health for everyone is fundamental to efforts to achieve global peace and security, which of course depends on full cooperation between individuals, community groups, nations, and countries in the world. A country's achievements in health promotion and protection have essential importance for all parties [11]. Therefore, knowledge and understanding of the concept of health for everyone is important, ensuring the achievement of the highest degree of health for all humans, as a whole. Forest therapy itself can be a valuable source of social support, contributing to an individual's overall well-being and quality of life. By facilitating social relationships, encouraging open communication, and creating shared experiences, forest therapy can be a powerful tool to increase social support and foster a sense of community. It can be argued that social support obtained through group activities can contribute to achieving the homeostasis of an individual's healthy triangle in improving physical and mental health while utilizing forest exposure as a medium to reduce stress and improve the body's immune system.

2. The benefit of forest therapy: reduce stress and anxiety

A meta-analysis examined the effect of exposure to natural environments on stress reduction and for stress management [12]. Similarly, other systematic reviews found the impact of forest therapy programs on stress reduction, examined the effectiveness of self-guided, and guided forest therapy in reducing stress levels, suggesting that both approaches can lead to positive outcomes [1, 6, 13]. Another study concluded that integrated indirect forest experiences can help increase positive emotions and reduce fatigue and stress levels during hemodialysis in chronic kidney failure patients. These findings recommend that forest therapy may be a useful tool to improve patients' quality of life [14].

In addition, forest therapy has benefits for reducing not only stress but also anxiety and depression. In fact, *Shinrin-yoku* can be effective in reducing mental health symptoms in the short term, particularly anxiety [15]. Its benefits are also supported by systematic reviews and meta-analyses aimed at summarizing the impact of forest therapy on depression and stress [16].

3. The benefit of immune system enhancement

The forest therapy programs have an impact on immune system enhancement. The immune function measurements such as NK cell count, NK cell cytotoxic activity, and cytotoxic effector molecules be effectively improved [17]. One study concludes that forest bathing trips have been found to increase NK activity, which is mediated by increases in NK cell number and intracellular anti-cancer protein levels. These findings suggest that forest bathing may have preventative effects against the onset and progression of cancer. The study also highlights the potential benefits of forest bathing for immune function and overall health [18].

The nature exposure supports immunological homeostasis and may offer promising strategies for therapeutic and preventive clinical use. However, there is a need to expand the field of study to a larger scale and larger study group, including different study populations and environments, and to standardize controls for confounding and environmental conditions [19]. A three-day session of bamboo forest therapy can have positive effects on the psychophysiology and immune system responses of male college students. These findings suggest that bamboo forest therapy may be a useful tool for improving physical and mental health, especially in urban populations [20].

However, it is still needed to do more randomized controlled trials (RCTs) on the impact of forest therapy on immune function, with larger and broader scale research, as well as more adequate cohort studies. Further research also includes different populations and research areas, to obtain standards for controlling confounding factors and environmental status, needed to strengthen the evidence supporting the use of forest therapy to improve immune function [17].

4. Reducing stress levels and improving immune function

The study explores the effects of forest therapy on the human psycho-neuro-endocrino-immune network, including its impact on the immune system. It discusses how forest therapy acts on the endocrine system to reduce stress hormone levels and its potential benefits for immune function. The results provide insights into the benefits of forest therapy on the immune system, highlighting its potential to improve immune activity and reduce stress levels [21].

A systematic review and meta-analysis aims to summarize the physio-psychological benefits of forest therapy, including its impact on stress reduction. This study reviews the physio-psychological benefits of forest therapy, including its impact on the immune system. It also discusses the role of biogenic volatile compounds in forests in improving human immunity and preventing infectious diseases [22]. The academic journals provide in-depth research and analysis on the positive effects of forest therapy on the immune system, stress reduction, and overall well-being. They offer precious awareness into the mechanisms by which forest therapy may improve immune function and contribute to better health outcomes [17].

5. Psychophysiological benefit

A comprehensive analysis of previous studies on the effects of forest therapy programs on stress reduction, by promoting relaxation, improving mood, and enhancing well-being across various populations, including children, adults, and older adults, was conducted [13]. The systematic review aims to examine the key findings of previous studies to explore how forest therapy programs impact stress reduction. The results indicate that forest therapy programs have a significant positive impact on stress reduction. The forest therapy programs can effectively reduce stress levels by promoting relaxation, improving mood, and enhancing overall well-being. They also noted that the effects of forest therapy programs on stress reduction are consistent across different populations, including children, adults, and older adults. Other studies have shown that in addition to stress reduction, forest therapy has been shown to provide many physical and mental health benefits, with additional benefits, such as promoting positive emotional change and social bonding through interactions with others [23]. Forest therapy can provide opportunities for self-reflection and introspection, leading to changes in one's mind and body, emotions, cognitive processes, and social interactions [24]. Likewise, the studies of where the physiological and psychosocial effects of forest therapy were shown to provide many physical and mental health benefits [6, 25].

The forest therapy has been found to have positive effects on both physical and mental health; however, the current research and its health outcomes involve various health indicators without unification of measure, highlighting the need for standardization of indicators to better understand the effects of forest therapy [25]. The forest therapy may be beneficial for health and well-being; however, the lack of high-quality studies limits the strength of the results, so more robust RCTs are warranted to establish the effectiveness of forest therapy for health encouragement and disease discouragement [26]. The indicators of the psychosocial and physiological effects of forest therapy involve spending time in the forest to promote physical and mental well-being as done in *Shinrin-yoku*, as well as forest walking in elderly populations [25, 27].

The study concluded that forest therapy may be beneficial for health promotion and disease prevention [26] through psychophysiological aspects, and this is reinforced by the study that concluded that forest walks have been shown to have positive effects on physical and mental health in the elderly population [27].

6. Worldwide popularity of forest therapy

Forest therapy has gained popularity globally as a means to promote human health and well-being through immersion in nature. The concept originated in Japan and has since been influenced by Japanese research in countries such as Korea, Taiwan, Malaysia, Australia, China, Sweden, Norway, and Germany.

Japan is the birthplace of forest therapy, with the term *Shinrin-yoku* created by the Ministry of Agriculture, Forestry and Fisheries of Japan in 1982. The meaning of this word is "breathing the atmosphere of the forest" or "bathing in the forest," and was proposed as a therapeutic means to counter the negative impacts of urbanization. Today, Japan has more than 60 forest therapy centers across the country, offering guidance and specialized pathways for therapeutic practices involving immersion in nature to enlarge mental and physical well-being [28].

Korea has been influenced by Japanese studies and has further developed its own forest therapy practices. Forest therapy in Korea is seen as an integrative tool for prevention and treatment of non-communicable diseases, with research focusing on its efficacy in cardiovascular rehabilitation [29]. Today, more than 37 forest therapy centers run by the central/local governments in Korea [30].

Taiwan has also been influenced by Japanese research and has developed its own forest therapy practices. Forest therapy in Taiwan is seen as a means to improve mental and physical health, with research focusing on its effects on stress reduction and overall well-being [31]. There are nine National Parks in Taiwan, and the country has a significant amount of forest cover, with 60% of its land area occupied by forests. However, the exact number of forest therapy centers in Taiwan is not specified in the provided information [32].

Malaysia has adopted forest therapy as a means to promote health tourism and well-being. Research in Malaysia has focused on the effects of forest therapy on mental health and stress reduction [32]. Malaysia has the potential to become a forest therapy reference center in Southeast Asia [33]. Additionally, there are studies and research being conducted on forest therapy in Malaysia, particularly focusing on its application for senior citizens' health care enhancement [34].

Australia has also adopted forest therapy, with the concept being introduced through the Japanese idea of *Shinrin-yoku.* Forest therapy in Australia is seen as a natural remedy to enhance general health and welfare, with research focusing on its effects on mental health and stress reduction [35].

Forest therapy in Australia is offered through various organizations, including:

- Forest Therapy Victoria works toward reconnecting people of all ages to nature for their health and well-being [36].

- The Institute of Forest Therapy, an Accredited Training Provider in Australia, Asia, and the Americas, offers forest therapy guide training workshops in Australia. It conducted a successful training workshop at Pallotti College in Victoria in September 2023 [37].

- In My Nature provides a self-paced online course on forest therapy, introducing participants to the history, research, science, and practices of Nature and Forest Therapy [38].

- Royal Botanic Gardens Victoria offers forest therapy sessions, allowing participants to reconnect with nature and spend time in the serene forested premises [39].

China has also been influenced by Japanese research and has developed its own forest therapy practices. Forest therapy in China is seen as an integrative tool for prevention and reception of non-communicable diseases, with research focusing on its efficacy in cardiovascular rehabilitation [40]. There are over 300 national forest rehabilitation and recreation centers in China planned to be constructed by 2022 to give standard forest therapy services at variance degrees and fulfill people's heightened necessity for a healthy lifestyle [41].

Sweden, Norway, and Germany have been involved in forest therapy research, with studies focusing on its effects on mental health and stress reduction [31].

The 2nd Global Summit of Science, Nature & Health in 2024 highlighted the practical application of scientific evidence in forest therapy, with speakers from various countries discussing the development of forest therapy in their respective countries [30].

7. Health triangle approach

Health Triangle Approach adopted WHO Constitution about "Health" that defines health as mental, physical, and social balance, also known as the health triangle [42]. Having a good balance in these three areas is very important for living a healthy lifestyle. This concept rules out that there is an interconnection between those three areas so that all need balances to achieve this. If one side of the triangle is too much—or not enough—then the other side of the triangle will change, thus producing an imbalance that disrupts homeostasis.

Health Triangle Approach may also look at it as "The Disease Triangle" that describes the interaction between pathogens, hosts, and the environment as a prerequisite for disease. This triangle can serve as a conceptual model that describes the factors that influence the development of an epidemic. Also included are examples of pathogens, hosts, and environmental factors that may influence their interactions and promote disease and thus the extent of disease epidemics.

The Triangle Approach to Health emphasizes that three favorable conditions – mental, physical, and social – as well as pathogen, host, and environmental factors, must coexist in balance to maintain health and prevent disease. This comprehensive framework helps to understand how environmental modalities, such as forest therapy, can contribute to overall health and well-being through dual effects on the host (including stress management and immune system support) and social interventions. By applying this approach, forest therapy can stabilize mental, physical, and social states and promote homeostasis between pathogen, host, and environment.

7.1 Mental health

Mental health stabilization is an important area in the Health Triangle Approach that must be considered, because a condition of psychological well-being allows persons to cope with life's tensions, maintain immune responses, perceive their capabilities, study and work excellently, and provide to their groups. These conditions are fundamental elements of human health and well-being that underlie humans' individual and collective capacities to make resolutions, construct alliances and bonds, and build the world in which we stay [43].

Mental health is a fundamental human right and essential for individual, group and socioeconomic growth. These states are continuous complex sequences (continuum), accomplished differently from one individual to other, with varying levels of distress and suffering, and potentially very unlike communal and objective outcomes. In every part of our lives, various individual, social, and structural factors can unite to preserve or weaken our mental health and change our situation on the mental health continuum [43].

Human psychological and biological factors, including emotional skills, drug use, and genetics, can make them more vulnerable to mental health problems. Exposure to adverse social, economic, geopolitical, and environmental conditions—including poverty, brutality, injustice, and environmental stress—also increases a person's risk of experiencing mental health disorders. These risks can occur at all stages of life but appear more easily and frequently in sensitive periods of human life development, especially in childhood and adolescence. Harsh parenting styles and physical punishment during development have a negative impact on the mental health of children and adolescents. Oppression or forcing their parents' will on them is a major risk factor for their mental health conditions. However, there are protective factors that also occur throughout our lives and function to strengthen mental health resilience, including social skills and attributes and emotional maturity as well as positive social interactions, quality education, decent work, a safe environment, and community cohesion [43].

Mental health dangers and safety components may be established in society at different degrees, and according to the Health Triangle Approach, these need to be localized and stabilized, then gradually eliminated. Individuals, families, and communities can experience local threats, while for the entire human population, global threats that also pose an increasing risk include; economic recession, pandemics, natural disasters, humanitarian disasters and displacement, conflict and war, and the increasing climate crisis. On the other hand, each of these risk factors and protective factors only has limited predictive power in terms of causing mental health disorders. Most people do not experience mental health disorder status even though they have been exposed to these risks, although many people whose risk factors are unknown actually experience mental health disorder status. However, the interacting determinants of mental health have a function and role in increasing or decreasing mental health status, causing stress and reducing the immune system [43].

7.2 Physical health

Physical health is how well our cells, tissues, organs, and body systems function. Each person's version of physical health is different and individually specific. A person can achieve his or her own definition of physical health, regardless of illness, disability, or age. The usual performing of an individual's body shows one dimension of total well-being, which is related to body growth, the functioning of the five senses, and movement, as well as how to care for the body and the intake of nutrients into the body [44].

The NZDF Health Hub provides physical health as everything we need to know about strengthening four pillars, that is, sleep (and recovery), nutrition, physical activity, and connection. Sleep is a simple and routine activity and is the most underestimated for improving health and performance. However, sleep actually really helps prevent excess weight gain, heart disease, and the emergence of disease. Humans, in fact all living creatures including cells, need a rest and recovery phase after stressful activities, both mentally and physically. The body needs sleep to allow and give time for it to repair itself and become fit, strengthen the immune system, and get ready for another day. Adequate and appropriate nutrition helps support performance, recovery, mental clarity, and overall mood, producing a better immune system as well. The body is like a car that can be driven well if it is filled with the right fuel. If we fill a racing car with regular petrol, it will be difficult for the car to compete against other racing cars filled with premium petrol, so it will most likely make an early pit stop. Quality nutrition provides fuel intake that suits the body's needs to work and recover, including reducing stress and reducing inflammation in the body due to injury, disease, and mental health problems. Little physical activity, lack of movement or exercise, will result in reducing the range of motion of the body's joints, resulting in joint dysfunction and pain. Because the body is designed to move, inactivity also contributes to a general decline in physical health, causing mental and physiological health disorders. Individuals who behave sedentary are at risk of experiencing various health problems including obesity, type 2 diabetes, cardiovascular disease, and mood disorders. However, people who exercise too much, overexercise, and are stressed can experience negative effects in the form of a body that is susceptible to fatigue and a weakened immune system. The human body will function best when it is in a situation of balance (homeostasis) of work, stress, and moderate physical activity, coupled with adequate rest. Note the advantage of physical activities; that is, they help maintain a healthy body weight, lower risk of heart disease, lower blood pressure, reduce risk of certain cancers, lower risk of type 2 diabetes, improve muscle strength and function, improve bone health and strength, help promote positive mental health, and reduce the risk of dementia. Keeping connected by always making connection with people is avoiding the loneliness [44].

Loneliness is the feeling of not having meaningful connections with other people in our life. It is possible to feel lonely in a crowd, or at work, and feel that we do not belong. A person may feel lonely even though in the eyes of others, they appear to have good social relationships and connections; for example, they have many professional work contacts without any deeper personal or psychological relationships other than that. There are times when we feel lonely, which may be because we withdraw from relationships with other people because we feel uncomfortable in groups. If connectivity causes anxiety and we start to avoid social relationships, we may experience social anxiety. Individuals who experience social anxiety often worry about what other people think about them, feel judged, or feel inadequate, so as a result, their comfort zone shrinks to the point where they feel isolated [44].

The Health Triangle Approach concerning physical health is keep anyone in balance states of their physical activities that supported by their four pillars.

7.3 Social health

Social health is an important aspect of overall well-being that points to an individual's capability to interact, form relationships, and function effectively within their social environment. The World Health Organization defines social health as "a state of well-being in which individuals realize their own ability to cope with the normal stresses of life, can work productively, and are able to contribute to society" [42]. The concept of social health has five key aspects [45]:

a. Social integration: evaluate the quality of a person's relationship with society and the community.

b. Social acceptance: evaluation of the qualities of others and the community.

c. Social contribution: evaluation of one's social worth and the extent to which one is a productive member of society.

d. Social actualization: evaluation of society's potential and trajectory.

e. Social coherence: perceptions of the quality, organization, and operation of the social world.

Maintaining good social health is essential for overall well-being, as it can positively impact physical and mental health, cognitive function, and quality of life. Numerous studies have demonstrated the importance of social health and its relationship with various health outcomes. A systematic review found that individuals with stronger social ties were 50% more likely to survive compared to those with weaker social ties [46]. Additionally, a longitudinal study showed that social relationships and social integration are associated with lower risk of mortality, better physical and mental health, and healthier behaviors [47].

Forest therapy has been shown to have a positive impact on the development of social health. There are physiological and psychological effects of viewing urban forest landscapes. The researchers found that spending time in forest environments can lead to improvements in various aspects of social health, including increased social connectedness, improved social competence, enhanced social participation, and increased social well-being [48].

8. Health triangle approach for forest therapy

The implementation of The Health Triangle Approach on Forest Therapy aims to reduce stress levels and improve the individual's immune system. Forest therapy may release a state of worrisome or mental tightness caused by a difficult situation. We should be able to experience stress in hard situations, because it is normal for us to perceive stressed in difficult conditions such as career audiences, educational tests, impracticable workloads, unstable work, or conflicts with family, friends, or coworkers. Stress decreases over time for most individuals, either as situations improve, or as they learn to cope emotionally. Stress tends to increase when events occur such as major economic crises, disease outbreaks, natural tragedies, conflicts, wars, and violence in society.

As a natural human response that drives us to overcome challenges and threats in our lives, stress in varying degrees and responses should be exposed to the natural touch of forest therapy. The duration and intensity of therapeutic exposure depends on the magnitude of the stress response that occurs individually, which makes a big difference to our overall well-being.

Forest therapy makes it easier for us to relax and cool a range of emotions, including anxiety and irritability. By walking in the forest, nature touches the senses, the sound of birds singing and the gurgling of flowing water, exposure to cool temperatures and wind, the smell of trees and soil restores the ability to concentrate, reduce headaches or other body pains, as well as upset stomach or trouble sleeping. This therapy can reverse loss of taste or eating more than usual, enhance chronic stress that can worsen preexisting health issues, and intercept increased use of alcohol, tobacco, and other substances.

Forest therapy can prevent stressful situations from causing or worsening mental strength states, most often worry and depression, that vital access to health care. If we hurt from a mental health state, it may be caused by tenacious symptoms of stress and start to impact our daily perform, involving at work or school. Everybody behaves differently to stressful circumstances and has their own ability to cope with stress, so stress symptoms vary individually. Thus, before conducting the therapy procedure, it is needed to make a short assessment.

The activities program on forest therapy affects both the mind (mental) and the body (physical) wellness, helps someone control stress by learning how to cope with it stress, can help us feel less overwhelmed, and support mental and physical well-being. As social health approach, forest therapy may create healthy and positive interpersonal relationships with one another (in a group setting), have close ties with family and friends, enjoy a sense of belonging to a group, and feel supported, appreciated, and loved. Having good social health helps people improve their emotional well-being and feel supported in their daily lives.

Forest therapy, as environmental exposure, enhances our mind and body, may control stress fluctuations well and remain functional, reduces stress and reduce difficulties in dealing with stress without needing professional help or from other people.

9. Forest therapy manages stress and improves our immune system

WHO's stress management guides what to do in things in times of stress, with the aim of equipping people with practical skills for dealing with stress. Individuals who have a few minutes each day are sufficient to practice self-help techniques with a guide. The guide can be used alone or accompanied by audio exercises. In this way, forest therapy (whether guided or unguided, individual or group, with a variety of innovative activities), as an environmental and social approach to the health triangle, can attract and maintain balance, and stabilize individual homeostasis, thereby maintaining health. Having a weekly schedule of forest therapy can help us use our time efficiently and feel more in control. Establish regular meal times, time with family members, exercise, and daily tasks during program activities [49].

Forest therapy may improve our immune system, because the program activities stimulate and affect us in getting sufficient sleep. This is essential for the body and mind. The efforts to improve sleep quality and relax and rejuvenate our bodies can help repair the effects of stress. If forest therapy is done in a group, it can improve aspects of our social health, as it enhances our social interactions with others, staying connected with family and friends and sharing concerns and feelings with people we trust. Individuals who can connect with others can improve their sense of security and their mood and help them reduce stress. Forest therapy should be done by walking, complemented by eating a healthy diet, because what we eat and drink can affect our health, so try to eat a balanced amount and quality of food and eat regularly. Drink enough fluids and eat plenty of fresh fruits and vegetables. If this therapy is done regularly, can help reduce stress. By walking during the activities of forest therapy regularly, it can help to reduce stress.

Promotional and preventive intervention efforts can be carried out by identifying key factors that determine individual, social, and structural mental health and then implementing interventions to reduce risk, build resilience, and build an environment that supports mental health. This Health Triangle Approach intervention can be designed for individuals, specific groups, or entire populations in forest therapy program activities.

Rebuilding mental health often requires movement beyond the health sector, so promotion and prevention activities through forest therapy should involve education, labor, justice, transportation, environment, housing, and welfare sectors, on an individual basis. Forest therapy can make a significant benefaction by incorporating advancement and constraint efforts into program activities and by supporting, establishing, and, where appropriate, raising the Health Triangle Approach.

As suicide prevention is a global priority and included in the Sustainable Development Goals [43], it is also may be targeted in forest therapy. Research shows that exposure to a forest environment can significantly reduce anxiety and depression, with participants reporting lower scores on mood state questionnaires following forest immersion [50].

Forest therapy ease to promote child and adolescent mental health, that may be pushed to be selected priorities required by policy and law, to promote and protect individual mental health, support parenting to provide nursing direction, implement school-based programs and improve the quality of online communities and environments. School-based social and emotional learning programs are one of the most effective promotional strategies for countries at all income levels. Efforts to promote and protect mental health in the workplace are an area of increasing interest and can also be supported through legislation, organizational strategies, manager training, and worker interventions.

On a national scale, efforts to strengthen mental health are critical to not only protect and improve the mental well-being of all people but also meet the needs of individuals with mental health status. Forest therapy should be implemented as a community-based, individualized mental health service option that is more accessible and acceptable than other mental health services and helps prevent human rights violations and provide better recovery outcomes for people with impaired mental health status. Community-based mental health services such as forest therapy should be provided through a network of interrelated services consisting of [43]:

- mental health services integrated within general health services, usually in general hospitals and through task sharing with nonspecialist service providers in primary health care;

- community mental health services that may involve community mental health care and teams, psychosocial rehabilitation points, drug and narcotic addiction services, peer support services, and living support services; and

- services that provide mental health services in social and non-health services, such as child protection, school health services, and prisons.

Countries that have limitations and large gaps in efforts to treat general mental health status, such as depression and anxiety, require innovative ways, such as forest therapy, to diversify and improve efforts to treat these conditions, in addition to nonspecialist psychological counseling therapy or digital self-help.

10. Conclusion and recommendation

The Health Triangle Approach provides a comprehensive framework for understanding the benefits of forest therapy, which can contribute to overall health and well-being through its positive impacts on stress management, immune system support, mental health promotion and prevention, physical fitness, social health, and the balance between host, pathogen, and environment. By adopting this approach, forest therapy can be an effective tool for improving individual and community health outcomes.

Author details

Hendro Prabowo[1] and Awal Prasetyo[2]*

1 Faculty of Psychology Gunadarma University, Depok, Indonesia

2 Faculty of Medicine, Diponegoro University, Semarang, Indonesia

*Address all correspondence to: awalpras@fk.undip.ac.id

References

[1] Seo JW, Kim K, Kim SG, Yi J, Shin W, Choi J, et al. Evaluation of the effectiveness of the elderly cognitive and exercise forest therapy program according to brain wave and autonomic nervous system parameters. Forests. 18 Jul 2024;**15**(7):1249. DOI: 10.3390/f15071249

[2] Satyawan VE, Rusdiana O, Latifah M. The role of forest therapy in promoting physical and mental health: A systematic review. IOP Conference Series: Earth and Environmental Science. 2022;**959**: 012027

[3] The University of British Columbia. The science of forest therapy. Available from: https://magazine.alumni.ubc.ca/2023/spring-2023/health-life-science/science-forest-therapy

[4] Arvay CG. Updating the biophilia hypothesis in the context of forest medicine. In: Kotte D et al., editors. International Handbook of Forest Therapy. Newcastle: Cambridge Scholars Publishing; 2019. pp. 21-32. ISBN: 1-5275-3955-5, ISBN13: 978-1-5275-3955

[5] Farkic J, Isailovic G, Taylor S. Forest bathing as a mindful tourism practice. Annals of Tourism Research Empirical Insights. 2021;**2**(2):1-9, 100028. DOI: 10.1016/j.annale.2021.100028

[6] Rajoo KS, Karam DS, Abdullah MZ. The physiological and psychosocial effects of forest therapy: A systematic review. Urban Forestry & Urban Greening. 2020;**54**:126744. DOI: 10.1016/j.ufug.2020.126744

[7] Barbiero G, Berto R. Biophilia as evolutionary adaptation: An onto- and phylogenetic framework for biophilic design. Frontiers in Psychology. 21 Jul 2021;**12**:1-13. Article 700709. DOI: 10.3389/fpsyg.2021.700709. PMID: 34367025; PMCID: PMC8334556

[8] Bowler DE, Buyung-Ali LM, Knight TM, et al. A systematic review of evidence for the added benefits to health of exposure to natural environments. BMC Public Health. 2010;**10**:456. DOI: 10.1186/1471-2458-10-456

[9] Jimenez MP, DeVille NV, Elliott EG, Schiff JE, Wilt GE, Hart JE, et al. Associations between nature exposure and health: A review of the evidence. International Journal of Environmental Research and Public Health. 2021;**18**(9):4790. DOI: 10.3390/ijerph18094790

[10] Kellert SR, Heerwagen J, Mador M. Biophilic Design: The Theory, Science and Practice of Bringing Buildings to Life. John Wiley & Sons; 2011

[11] World Health Organization (WHO). WHO remains firmly committed to the principles set out in the preamble to the constitution. Available from: https://www.who.int/about/governance/constitution

[12] Yao W, Zhang X, Gong Q. The effect of exposure to the natural environment on stress reduction: A meta-analysis. Urban Forestry & Urban Greening. 2021;**57**:126932. DOI: 10.1016/j.ufug.2020.126932

[13] Zhang Y, Feng L, Duan W. The impact of forest therapy programs on stress reduction: A systematic review. Forests. 2023;**14**(9):1851. DOI: 10.3390/f14091851

[14] Kang H, Chae Y. Effects of integrated indirect forest experience on emotion,

fatigue, stress and immune function in hemodialysis patients. International Journal of Environmental Research and Public Health. 2021;**18**(4):1701. DOI: 10.3390/ijerph18041701

[15] Kotera Y, Richardson M, Sheffield D. Effects of *Shinrin-Yoku* (forest bathing) and nature therapy on mental health: A systematic review and meta-analysis. International Journal of Mental Health and Addiction. 2022;**20**:337-361. DOI: 10.1007/s11469-020-00363-4

[16] Yeon PS, Jeon JY, Jung MS, Min GM, Kim GY, Han KM, et al. Effect of forest therapy on depression and anxiety: A systematic review and meta-analysis. International Journal of Environmental Research and Public Health. 2021;**18**(23):12685. DOI: 10.3390/ijerph182312685

[17] Chae Y, Lee S, Jo Y, Kang S, Park S, Kang H. The effects of forest therapy on immune function. International Journal of Environmental Research and Public Health. 2021;**18**(16):8440. DOI: 10.3390/ijerph18168440

[18] Li Q. Effect of forest bathing trips on human immune function. Environmental Health and Preventive Medicine. 2010;**15**(1):9-17. DOI: 10.1007/s12199-008-0068-3

[19] Andersen L, Corazon SSS, Stigsdotter UKK. Nature exposure and its effects on immune system functioning: A systematic review. International Journal of Environmental Research and Public Health. 2021;**18**(4):1416. DOI: 10.3390/ijerph18041416

[20] Lyu B, Zeng C, Xie S, Li D, Lin W, Li N, et al. Benefits of a three-day bamboo forest therapy session on the psychophysiology and immune system responses of male college students. International Journal of Environmental Research and Public Health. 2019;**16**(24):4991. DOI: 10.3390/ijerph16244991

[21] Li Q, Kawada T. Effect of forest therapy on the human psycho-neuro-endocrino-immune network. Nihon Eiseigaku Zasshi. 2011;**66**(4):645-650. Japanese. DOI: 10.1265/jjh.66.645

[22] Yi Y, Seo E, An J. Does forest therapy have physio-psychological benefits? A systematic review and meta-analysis of randomized controlled trials. International Journal of Environmental Research and Public Health. 2022;**19**(17):10512. DOI: 10.3390/ijerph191710512

[23] Kim JG, Shin WS. Forest therapy alone or with a guide: Is there a difference between self-guided forest therapy and guided forest therapy programs? International Journal of Environmental Research and Public Health. 2021;**18**(13):6957

[24] Shin W-S, Seong I-K, Kim J-G. Psychological benefits of self-guided forest healing program using campus forests. Forests. 2023;**14**(2):336. DOI: 10.3390/f14020336

[25] Chun H-r, Choi Y-Y, Cho I, Nam H-k, Kim G, Park S, et al. Indicators of the psychosocial and physiological effects of forest therapy: A systematic review. Forests. 2023;**14**(7):1407. DOI: 10.3390/f14071407

[26] Oh B, Lee KJ, Zaslawski C, et al. Health and well-being benefits of spending time in forests: Systematic review. Environmental Health and Preventive Medicine. 2017;**22**:71. DOI: 10.1186/s12199-017-0677-9

[27] Piva G, Caruso L, Gómez AC, Calzolari M, Visintin EP, Davoli P, et al. Effects of forest walking on

physical and mental health in elderly populations: A systematic review. Reviews on Environmental Health. 2022;**39**(1):121-136. DOI: 10.1515/reveh-2022-0093

[28] Griffiths B. How forest therapy changed my relationship with the great outdoors. Available from: https://www.polar.com/blog/forest-therapy/

[29] Lee J, Shin WS. Forest therapy in Korea. In: Kotte D et al., editors. International Handbook of Forest Therapy. Newcastle: Cambridge Scholars Publishing; 2019. ISBN: 1-5275-3955-5, ISBN13: 978-1-5275-3955-6

[30] Forest Therapy Hub. Won Sop Shin and the Korean Public Policy on Forests for Happiness, Health and Welfare. Available from: https://foresttherapyhub.com/won-sop-shin-and-the-korean-public-policy-on-forests-for-happiness-health-and-welfare/

[31] Gobster PH, Schultz CL, Kruger LE, Henderson JR. Forest therapy trails: A conceptual framework and scoping review of research. Forests. 2022;**13**(10):1613. DOI: 10.3390/f13101613

[32] National Park Service Ministry of the Interior. Purify the mind—Nature therapy@National Park. Available from: https://www.nps.gov.tw/np-quarterly.html?catid=64&id=621&ls=1&view=en detail

[33] University Putra Malaysia. Malaysia has Potential to be a Forest Therapy Reference Centre in Southeast Asia. UPM; 2024. Available from: https://www.upm.edu.my/news/malaysia_has_potential_to_be_a_forest_therapy_reference_centre_in_southeast_asia-61336

[34] Karam DS, Rajoo KS. Forest therapy in Malaysia. In: Kotte D et al., editors. International Handbook of Forest Therapy. Cambridge Scholars Publishing; 2019

[35] Joachim SV. Forest therapy in Australia. In: Kotte D et al., editors. International Handbook of Forest Therapy. Cambridge Scholars Publishing; 2019

[36] Forest Therapy Victoria. Health and wellbeing in nature. Available from: https://www.foresttherapyvictoria.com.au

[37] INFTA. Forest therapy guide training in Australia. Available from: https://infta.net/forest-therapy-guide-training-in-australia/

[38] In My Nature. Forest therapy guide training in Australia. Available from: http://inmynature.life/shinrin-yoku-australia/training/

[39] Royal Botanic Gardens Victoria. Forest therapy at Melbourne gardens. Available from: https://www.rbg.vic.gov.au/melbourne-gardens/what-s-on-melbourne/forest-therapy/

[40] Liu L, Ye B, Zhang Z, Gao Y. The origin and development of Chinese forest therapy. In: Kotte D et al., editors. International Handbook of Forest Therapy. Cambridge Scholars Publishing; 2019

[41] Zhang Z, Wang P, Gao Y, Ye B. Current development status of forest therapy in China. Healthcare. 2020;**8**(1):61

[42] World Health Organization. Constitution of the World Health Organization. In: World Health Organization: Handbook of Basic Documents. 1952. pp. 3-20

[43] World Health Organization (WHO). Mental health. Available from: https://

www.who.int/news-room/fact-sheets/detail/mental-health-strengthening-our-response/?gad_source=1&gclid=Cj0KCQjwtZK1BhDuARIsAAy2VztR4KS5jlvNdvb_YaW20f6ZtwiGSMjmibr-5lGLqCelpHeu-M71pi0aAp0BEALw_wcB

[44] Defence Health Hub. What is physical health. Available from: https://health.nzdf.mil.nz/your-health/body/physical-health-and-fitness/what-is-physical-health/

[45] Keyes CL, Social well-being. Social Psychology Quarterly. 1998:121-140

[46] Holt-Lunstad J, Smith TB, Layton JB. Social relationships and mortality risk: A meta-analytic review. PLoS Medicine. 2010;**7**(7):e1000316

[47] Umberson D, Karas MJ. Social relationships and health: A flashpoint for health policy. Journal of Health and Social Behavior. 2010;**51**(1_suppl):S54-S66

[48] Tsunetsugu Y, Lee J, Park BJ, Tyrväinen L, Kagawa T, Miyazaki Y. Physiological and psychological effects of viewing urban forest landscapes assessed by multiple measurements. Landscape and Urban Planning. 2013;**113**:90-93

[49] World Health Organization (WHO). Stress: How can I manage stress. Available from: https://www.who.int//news-room/questions-and-answers/item/stress/?gad_source=1&gclid=Cj0KCQjwtZK1BhDuARIsAAy2VzurZCv4PNoJN0L5nEBuEfKE2uQNTGrwzXonRdPjv_0WNCpErUptIQgaAu63EALw_wcB

[50] Le Gear K, Carlin C, Flaherty GT. Deep roots: Realising the public health benefits of exposure to forest environments. Advances in Integrative Medicine. 2023;**10**(2):86-88

Chapter 4

Green Practices and Innovations Oriented toward a Lifestyle Connected with Nature

Erika Loučanová and Martina Nosáľová

Abstract

Globalization has led to an increase in the popularity of alternative medicine, particularly those that emphasize living a natural lifestyle. In addition to the necessities of life, such as food, nature also provides us with nature medical needs. These in a different character are widely used in modern as well as in traditional folk medicine. These methods may be considered innovative green practices since they are not customary in the regions where they occur. The aim of the paper is to find out Slovakian society's perceptions on various forms of alternative medicine that represent a lifestyle connected to nature, such as forest wellness, phytotherapy, regenerative environmental design, and so on. The examined object was observed using the Kano model on a randomized sample of Slovakian respondents. The results confirmed that different types of alternative medicine representing a lifestyle connected to nature are used rather than disease prevention or elimination of nongreen procedures. Innovations in health maintenance and ecological practices focused on a lifestyle connected to nature can have a positive impact on people's lives.

Keywords: green practice, innovation, nature, complementary and alternative medicine, attitude, Kano model

1. Introduction

Throughout human history, there has been discussion about the link between humans and nature. The concept of being connected to nature has emerged as a significant transdisciplinary subject of research in more recent times [1].

Nature connectedness is understood as the degree to which a person possesses the quality of feeling a connection to the natural environment as a possible way to foster emotional connections [2, 3]. Essentially, the terms "nature connectedness" and "love for nature" relate to people's deep affection for the natural world and its environs. These connections are typically characterized, for example, by people's feelings, beliefs, and behavioral tendencies toward the natural world [3]. The degree to which a person feels a connection to the nature can be a good indicator of their love of the nature leading to behavior that is helpful to the environment, such as buying green products [3]. Consumer interest for natural products has increased in the last several years. The authors describe this kind of drive as biophilia, or the love of nature. Declaring a product's natural state is in line with current consumer tendencies toward sustainable and healthful consumption [4].

As environmental issues have become more prevalent, people's concern for the environment has expanded significantly. These issues have a variety of effects on consumer behavior, including choices and purchase patterns [5]. Apart from the consumers themselves, it is exactly the environment that influences the variety of product selection habits. Similarly, one's decision-making regarding goods purchases may be impacted also themselves (their family) or the environment. In addition, each individual consumer may have different variables influencing their decision on purchase, such as disparities in their gender, age, education, job, as well as monthly spending on food and beverage goods [6].

Based on the above, there is a new term in the area of interest—lifestyle—having a significant effect on customer purchase decision. It is a newer concept as the pattern in which people live and use or spend money and time [7]. Due to the changes in people lifestyles, the access to environment, wildlife, and green places around us has been restricted. According to the data of United Nations [6], currently, 55% of people on Earth reside in cities; by 2050, that number is expected to rise to 68%. Actual changes in lifestyle manifested in the form of the apartment culture of housing, smaller and dense communities, as well as increased use of television, internet, and mobile phones worsened the situation [8].

Public health and environmental sustainability present two of the most significant global challenges of the twenty-first century [9], while, for example, the reference [10] points out on an increasing recognition that these two challenges are interconnected. Numerous health- and sustainability-related outcomes are linked to both psychological connectivity and physical contact with nature. There are now six official pillars of lifestyle medicine, and there is actually growing evidence that daily exposure to nature and fresh air is essential for optimizing overall physical and mental health [11]. It was discovered that particular forms of engagement with nature, together with individual variations in nature connectivity, had distinct associations with elements of health, happiness, and pro-environmental actions [9]. This is also confirmed by study [12], where it is demonstrated that spending time in nature improves mental health in addition to its physical health benefits, or even the reference [13] that points out that interactions with the countryside are beneficial to the physical and psychological health of young people, as well as for their social, cognitive, and educational development. Even with proof of nature's advantages, people are spending less time in the nature [8].

In recent years, therefore, more attention has been paid not only to eco-innovations focusing on economic but also to environmental and social aspects. In combining these three aspects toward sustainability, in terms of reducing overall emissions or existing environmental burdens and health risks, the overall ideas of healthy lifestyles and sustainable consumption have begun to be promoted [14, 15].

Because of globalization, various types of alternative medicine focusing on lifestyles connected to nature are gaining popularity around the world. Lifestyle medicine is also mentioned more often. Many consider lifestyle medicine to be a relatively new subspecialty, although it has been practiced for 1000s of years. Unlike conventional medicine, the focus of lifestyle medicine is not on the treatment of chronic diseases but rather on their prevention [16].

Along with having greater knowledge and expressing a poorer state of health, most people who use alternative medicine seem to be doing so primarily because they find these healthcare options to be more in line with their personal values, beliefs, and philosophical orientations toward life and health rather than because they are not satisfied with conventional medicine [17, 18]. Numerous studies' findings indicate that a sizable and potentially rising segment of the population uses complementary or alternative medicine (CAM) nowadays [19]. According to the US National Institutes of Health [20], CAM is "a group of diverse medical and health care systems, practices, and products that are not presently considered to be part of conventional medicine." Complementary medicine refers to therapy used in combination with conventional medicine, while alternative medicine is a term for medicine used instead of it. The NIH divide CAM into 5 groups: alternative medical systems (e.g., homeopathy, Chinese medicine, and Ayurvedic medicine), mind-body interventions (e.g., meditation, mental training, and art therapy), biologically based therapies (e.g., herbs and nutritional supplements), manipulation therapies (e.g., chiropractic and massage), and energy therapies (e.g., healing). Nevertheless, with the increasing variety of alternative medicine focuses, the number of subgroups differs too.

An increased level of public's utilization of herbal products is causing significant emerging of economic benefits. The key reason is that people are becoming more proactive about their health and looking for alternative forms of treatment to maintain it [21]. Also, non-wood forest products are collected or harvested for commercial and medical purposes from forests. These plants can be diversified into wild food plants, medicinal and aromatic plants, bulbous plants, mushrooms, dye plants, and honey. People buy medicinal plants mostly for the treatment of respiratory system and digestive system diseases, and the demand is generally high in winter and autumn. The most important factor affecting the purchasing preferences of consumers is freshness. The consumers mostly buy the medicinal plants from herbalists [22]. Furthermore, new forms of natural therapies are becoming more and more popular. The scope of health benefits of forest bathing/forest therapy and of time in nature has been increasingly documented over four decades of research. One powerful advantage of Forest Therapy is that while it enhances the well-being of participants, it also expands our awareness of participating in a cooperative, reciprocal ecosystem, which we can emulate and advance in our healthcare delivery systems [12].

Making decisions on a course of treatment and therapy can be challenging and complex, requiring patients to weigh all possible physical and psychological side effects [23]. Psychological considerations also impact the decision of treatment [24]. Patients who base their treatment decisions on their personal views may find it more difficult to choose a course of treatment. Personal beliefs are especially important when there is a lot of uncertainty about the treatment's long-term effects [23, 25, 26].

Decision-making processes play an important role in the field of medicine. Healthcare professionals make various decisions on a constant basis. These decisions are related to different matters, such as the type of diagnostics or intervention, modification of the standard procedures, or how make a treatment more effective [27]. Decisions in healthcare can be particularly strained, involving a complex web of diagnostic and therapeutic uncertainties, patient preferences, values, and costs [28]. Very frequently, these decisions have serious outcomes and can result in possible financial or human harm. Decision-making in the area of healthcare has specific features [27]; paramedic decision-making situations are characterized by complexity and time pressure [29].

Consumers' concern for the environment is growing as a result of the modern world. Their buying habits have started to reflect these worries, and environmental consciousness has given rise to a new market category known as "green consumers."

Since not every customer is equally environmentally conscious, consumer segmentation is required. In the following section, we focus on the possible link between environmental consumers' segmentation models and their interest in different types of medicines.

The NMI National Marketing Institute [30] has developed the LOHAS, Lifestyle of Health and Sustainability segmentation, model, which places consumers into one of five groups depending on their awareness and involvement in environmental issues as follows: LOHAS consumers, Naturalites, Drifters, Conventionals, and Unconcerneds. Although we focused on the LOHAS model when we proposed the green consumers segmentation model, we also considered another segmentation studies as Ottman's segmentation [31] as well as Ziaei-Bideh and Namakshenas-Jahromi's model [32]. Our proposed model implements the categorization and characteristics of these segments and provides its own perspective on segmentation model of environmental lifestyle. Market segments there can be named and characterized as follows:

LOHAS consumers—they are environmental stewards who use green products frequently, are socially conscious, and are motivated to preserve the environment. They take action and inspire others to follow suit in order to maintain the well-being of the earth and themselves.

- *Resource conservers*—they hate waste. They prefer reusable packaging, sustainable clothing. They recycle and reuse and avoid overpackaged products. They are responsible users of energies and resources.

- *Animal lovers*—they are concerned about animals; they treat them responsibly; their love for animals is reflected in their attitudes toward products; they are likely to be vegetarian or vegan.

These consumer groups present the features by which we can name and classify them by term of Ziaei-Bideh and Namakshenas-Jahromi model [32] as *Intense greens.*

Naturalites—they base the majority of their purchasing decisions on the advantages for their own health. They are not as involved in planetary health, despite their interest in environmental protection, which is mostly motivated by concerns for their own health.

- *Outdoor enthusiasts*—they spend their free time in nature, camping, and their love for nature is manifested in their behavior and preferences; they seek to minimize the impact of their recreational activities. When shopping, they look for sustainable labels on their products; they are also likely to purchase products from recycled materials.

- *Health fanatics*—they worry about the impact of products and behavior on their health; they prefer organic foods and natural cosmetics; they are well-informed and educated about the impact on their health.

Drifters—they are motivated by the latest trends; these consumers' commitment to any issue, including sustainability, is constantly shifting. General population in NMI defined consumer segments) youngest segment; Drifters are more likely to view price as a barrier to green living.

Conventionals—they are not very concerned about the environment because they are more motivated by frugal living and pragmatism than by pure environmental benefits. On the other hand, they do participate in certain environment-related activities, like energy conservation and recycling.

These consumer groups present the features by which we can name and classify them by term of Ziaei-Bideh and Namakshenas-Jahromi model [32] as *Potential greens.*

Unconcerneds—they represent the portion of the population that exhibits no sense of environmental responsibility.

These consumer groups present the features by which we can name and classify them by term of Ziaei-Bideh and Namakshenas-Jahromi model [31] as *Browns.*

Subsequently, **Table 1** provides an overview of our proposed segmentation model of environmental life style of consumers, where their characteristics according to green behavior in relation to attitudes toward different types of medicine, as well as possible ways of marketing appeal of the consumer segment are present. Innovations in health maintenance and ecological practices focused on a lifestyle connected to nature can have a positive impact on people's lives.

As it is evident from **Table 1**, consumers' interest in the environment is related to their daily behavior, buying habits, as well as attitudes and preferences to specific product and service to different category of medicine and models to lifestyle, too. In our study, we focus on the possible link between environmental consumers' segmentation models and their interest in different types of medicines. The aim of the paper is to find out Slovakian society's perceptions on various forms of alternative medicine that represent a lifestyle connected to nature, such as forest spa, phytotherapy, regenerative environmental design, and so on in comparison to the conventional medicine. Using the KANO model, we want to find out the level of attractiveness, mandatory occurrence, or indifference in relation to various different types of medicine.

2. Methodology

The Kano model technique is used to distinguish conventional medicine from complementary and alternative medicine from the perspective of social perception [14]. This allows us to identify all the relevant requirements of individuals. Using the Kano model, we are able to examine how an individual's unique needs are dependent on both conventional and alternative treatments in a nonlinear and asymmetric dependence. This is based on the individual and cumulative satisfaction with the variables under observation.

The basic steps of the Kano model provide the foundation for a methodical approach to identifying the relevant individual requirements of conventional and alternative medicine.

The first phase entails identifying the fundamental categories of alternative medicine that have been noticed based on the literature: phytotherapy (herbalism),[1]

[1] "Phytotherapy is the study of the use of extracts of natural origin as medicines or health-promoting agents. Phytotherapy medicines differ from plant-derived medicines in standard pharmacology. Where standard pharmacology isolates an active compound from a given plant, phytotherapy aims to preserve the complexity of substances from a given plant with relatively less processing."

Authors' models to lifestyle	**LOHAS**	**Ziaei-Bideh and Namakshenas-Jahromi**	**Ottman**	**Characteristics**	**Category of medicine**	**Ways to appeal the consumer segment**
Types	LOHAS consumers	Intense greens	Resource conservers Animal lovers	• Values-driven (by personal and planetary health) • Passionate recyclers, energy and water savers • They use gentle technologies • Animal and nature lovers • Green, healthy, and socially conscious product buyers • They seek out companies who practice corporate social responsibility	• Phytotherapy • Aromatherapy • Flower therapy - or other natural, alternative medicine • Regenerative environmental design • Forest wellness • Homeopathy • In necessary cases, conventional medicine	• Highlight the economical, long-lasting, and reusability benefits of products • Offer services that enable them to recycle, compost, and save energy • Conduct targeted marketing campaigns (for example, helping animals, advertising in magazines focused on the environment, animals, etc.) • CSR development
	Naturalites		Outdoor enthusiasts Health fanatics	• Spending leisure time in nature and practice sports in nature • Driven by personal health and wellness and adhere to a healthy lifestyle • They are looking for natural and organic foods, natural cosmetics • - they are loyal to those companies/ brands who practice credible CSR	• Forest wellness • Flower therapy • Aromatherapy • Phytotherapy • Or other natural, alternative medicine • Regenerative environmental design • Homeopathy • In necessary cases, conventional medicine	• Focus on organic aspects, health benefits, trust, transparency, and natural ingredients • Cross-promote with organic foods companies or a nontoxic cleaning product - conduct a joint promotion with national parks or manufacturers of boots, reusable bottles, and trail mix snacks • CSR development
Authors' models to lifestyle	LOHAS	Ziaei-Bideh and Namakshenas-Jahromi	Ottman	Characteristics	Category of medicine	Ways to appeal the consumer segment

DOI: http://dx.doi.org/10.5772/intechopen.1006137

Authors' models to lifestyle	**LOHAS**	**Ziaei-Bideh and Namakshenas-Jahromi**	**Ottman**	**Characteristics**	**Category of medicine**	**Ways to appeal the consumer segment**
Types	Drifters			• They are driven by trends • They are engaged in sustainability although their behaviors are not deeply rooted • They are price-sensitive	• Depending on current trends, they lean toward individual types of alternative and conventional medicine	• Focus on trends in sustainability • Emphasize the benefits of sustainability and the economic, long-term, and reusable benefits of the products • Offer services that are in line with current sustainability trends; targeted marketing campaigns focused mainly on price
	Conventionals	Potential greens		• This is practical segment • Does not have green attitudes but does have some "municipal" environmental behaviors such as recycling, energy conservation, and other similar behaviors • This segment's behavior is driven more by cost savings or a desire to waste less than by environmental consciousness	• Conventional medicine complemented by various types of alternative, or natural medicine	• Emphasize the benefits of sustainability and the economic, long-term, and reusable benefits of the products • Education • Conduct targeted marketing campaigns (for example, environmental education activities, subsidy schemes for introducing ecological solutions, etc.)
Authors' models to lifestyle	LOHAS	Ziaei-Bideh and Namakshenas-Jahromi	Ottman	Characteristics	Category of medicine	Ways to appeal the consumer segment

Authors' models to lifestyle	LOHAS	Ziaei-Bideh and Namakshenas-Jahromi	Ottman	Characteristics	Category of medicine	Ways to appeal the consumer segment
Types	Unconcerneds	Browns		• Not environmentally conscientious at all; tendencies to have negative attitudes about the environment • Nongreen behaviors • Altruistic, biospheric, and religious values are very low, and they are egoistic consumers - low knowledge or no interest in the environment and social issues mainly because they do not have time or resources	• Conventional medicine, which can be supplemented with various types of alternative, or natural medicine	• Education • Conduct targeted marketing campaigns (for example, environmental education activities, subsidy schemes for introducing ecological solutions, etc.)

Source: Developed by the authors based on the literature used.

Table 1.
Segmentation models to lifestyle consumers.

aromatherapy,[2] homeopathy,[3] flower therapy,[4] regenerative environmental design,[5] and forest wellness[6] [33–40]. The mentioned forms of complementary and alternative medicine will be examined compared to conventional medicine.

A questionnaire with positive and negative statements is created based on the types of conventional and alternative medicine that have been generated. The questionnaire is designed to gather responses from consumers on a Likert scale, which ranges from strongly disagree to neutral, partially agree to strongly disagree.

The fundamental technique for determining each person's unique needs is questioning; in our study, it is used as a multifaceted approach that aims to acquire and collect primary data regarding people's behaviors and attitudes toward different types of medicine. Because of the relevance of the research, it is necessary to count minimal sample of respondents (n) according to the formula:

$$n = \frac{z^2 * p * (1 - p) + e^2}{e^2 + z^2 * p * \frac{(1-p)}{N}} \tag{1}$$

where n—population size; e—permissible margin of error; p—variance in %; z—confidence level.

The process of questioning and obtaining the necessary attitudes of respondents is followed by the creation of KANO database. The Kano model cross rule is used to analyze form of individual statement to the positively and negatively asked questions separately. Based on this evaluation, the attitude specific to analyzed type of medicine is founded. This approach classifies the observed types of medicine from the

---

[2] "Aromatherapy uses plant materials and aromatic plant oils, including essential oils, and other aromatic compounds, for the purpose of altering one's mood, cognitive, psychological, or physical well-being."

[3] "Homeopathy is a system of alternative medicine based on his doctrine of like cures like, a claim that a substance that causes the symptoms of a disease in healthy people would cure similar symptoms in sick people."

[4] Flower therapy is "solutions of brandy and water—the water containing extreme dilutions of flower material developed by Edward Bach, an English homeopath, in the 1930s. Bach claimed that dew found on flower petals retain imagined healing properties of that plant."

[5] "Regenerative environmental design is an emerging discipline of sustainable architecture that focuses on building interrelationships between diverse entities, design, processes, and the responsibilities of various stakeholders at numerous levels. It broadens and utilizes knowledge on ecosystem services and living habitats. It is based on the core concepts of living systems thinking to create a constructed environment in which humans and nature may coevolve and mutually prosper. Regenerative design in the built environment largely focuses on facilitating healthy processes and flows within one focal scale of a system without catalyzing change at larger scales. The regenerative design takes into account not only the architecture but also the people, culture, and other activities involved. According to linked literature, the function of regenerative design requires a connection and linkage between the place's historical, cultural, ecological, and economic patterns, as well as a joint vision for a better future."

[6] The forest wellness or bathing, also known as Japanese practice of shinrin-yoku, not only has become a new wellness trend but also has the potential to offer tourists profoundly immersive experiences. Numerous studies have examined the positive effects of forest bathing, focusing primarily on its health benefits; forest bathing alludes to its latent capacity to provide a profoundly mindful experience and aims to elevate this practice within the tourism discourse. The purpose of wellness tourism is to promote physical and mental health and relaxation. A wellness trip may facilitate a genuine lifestyle transformation.

		Negative conceived question				
		Strong agreement	**Partial agreement**	**Neutral stance**	**Partial disagreement**	**Strong disagreement**
Positive conceived question	Strong agreement	Q	A	A	A	O
	Partial agreement	R	I	I	I	M
	Neutral stance	R	I	I	I	M
	Partial disagreement	R	I	I	I	M
	Strong disagreement	R	R	R	R	Q

Table 2.
KANO model to assess the needs of respondents [14].

viewpoint of social perception into: must be (M), one-dimensional (O), attractive (A), reverse (R), indifferent (I), and questionable (Q) (**Table 2**).

According to several references [41, 42], individual attitude categories influencing the satisfaction of respondents in relation to the different types of medicine studied can be characterized as follows:

Must be (M) requirements are seen as natural and are taken for granted by people. They can be categorized as primary or basic, and people only pay attention to them when they are not met. Their identification is crucial primarily because, while fulfilling these needs will affect people's satisfaction, people will notice deficits and nonfulfillment right away, leaving them unhappy, unsatisfied.

One-dimensional requirements (O) are those characteristics of the product that, when met, cause people to be content; conversely, when these requirements are not met, people become dissatisfied. In other words, the more often these criteria are met, the more satisfied people are. On the other hand, people do not always demand one-dimensional needs, unlike mandatory (must-be) requirements. Individual satisfaction and the fulfillment of these requirements are directly correlated linearly. Attractive requirements (A) are those, which have a clear effect on the satisfaction of individuals, because they do not expect them. In case that these requirements are not fulfilled, it will not result in dissatisfaction of individuals.

Reverse requirements (R), sometimes referred to as the exact opposite in some studies [43], are characteristics of a product that cause consumers to respond contradictorily.

Referred to as insignificant requirements, *indifferent requirements (I)* are those attributes that are not essential for customers and whose fulfillment or nonfulfillment has no impact on the level of satisfaction or dissatisfaction expressed by the customers.

Questionable or unclear requirements (Q) express uncertain results, which are connected to either improperly formulated questions or consumers' misinterpretation of the questions.

The individual requirements of the selected medicine types are then categorized and expressed as a percentage, with the category with the highest percentage identifying the particular category of the observed medicine type. The percentage of all observed requirements of the examined quantity of a particular medicine is represented by the maximum value requirement (%) of the recognized specific category.

Using Microsoft Excel software, the correlation coefficient—which measures the degree of dependency between two quantitative variables—will be employed to ascertain the dependence of individual Kano model results. Its value clarifies how these two variables' values are changing at the same time. The positive values means that they are changing together in one direction; the negative value means that they are changing in opposite direction, and the zero value means that they are changing independent of each other. Its value ranges from −1 to 1. If the absolute value of correlation coefficient in psychological research is below 0.1, it shows trivial dependency; if the value is in the range from 0.1 to 0.3, it shows small dependency; the range from 0.3 to 0.5 shows moderate dependency, and the value above 0.5 shows heavy dependency [44].

3. Results and discussion

Globalization has led to an increase in the popularity of alternative medicine, particularly those that emphasize living a natural lifestyle. The overall ideas of healthy lifestyles and sustainable consumption have begun to be promoted. Consequently, making decisions on a course of treatment and therapy can be challenging and complex, affected by many factors. Our study examine the attitudes of respondents in Slovakia toward conventional, complementary and alternative medicine. In order to observe the diversity of attitudes on the scale of positive and negative perception, KANO model was used. The KANO model has the potential to monitor the impact of attributes on individuals in terms of satisfaction that is from the viewpoint of interaction between the inner and outer psychological motives [45].

Based on the aforementioned, the Kano questionnaire was created, and a random research was conducted in Slovakia using these questionnaires. The questionnaire survey was intended for the population of Slovakia, while the total sample consisted of 275 respondents. For the calculation of the sample, we used the total population in Slovakia for the year 2023 with the number of 5,424,687 inhabitants [46], with a confidence level of 95%, a variance of 50%, and a permissible margin of error of 7%.

For the relevance of the surveys, we calculated the sample of respondents according to the following calculation:

$$n = \frac{(z^2 \times p \times (1-p)) + e^2}{e^2 + z^2 \times p \times \frac{(1-p)}{N}} = \frac{(95^2 \times 50 \times (1-50)) + 7^2}{7^2 + 95^2 \times 50 \times \frac{(1-50)}{5\ 424687}} = 197 \tag{2}$$

where population size (N): 5,424,687; permissible margin of error in % (e): 7; variance in % (p): 50; confidence level in % (z): 95; sample size needed (n): 197.

Based on the results of the survey and using the KANO cross rule, respondents in Slovakia indicate the following attitudes to different types of medicine (**Table 3**).

As can be seen from **Table 3**, respondents show an indifferent attitude for all types of medicine surveyed, which is the most frequently represented requirement for respondents in Slovakia. Individual types of medicine, either conventional or alternative types of medicine, do not have a significant influence on the individuals in society. Nevertheless, the crucial fact is that primary results of the survey, however, do not take into consideration other significant influence, for example morbidity of

Research parameters	Frequency	Requirements					
		Must-be	Attractive	One dimensional	Reverse	Indifferent	Questionable
Conventional medicine	Absolutely	40	15	24	22	171	3
	Relatively	14.55	5.45	8.73	8.00	62.18	1.09
Regenerative environmental design	Absolutely	28	59	20	31	130	7
	Relatively	10.18	21.45	7.27	11.27	47.27	2.55
Phytotherapy	Absolutely	8	85	22	36	110	14
	Relatively	2.91	30.91	8.00	13.09	40.00	5.09
Aromatherapy	Absolutely	15	56	24	24	150	6
	Relatively	5.45	20.36	8.73	8.73	54.55	2.18
Homeopathy	Absolutely	13	31	3	50	165	13
	Relatively	4.73	11.27	1.09	18.18	60.00	4.73
Flower therapy	Absolutely	31	17	8	56	158	5
	Relatively	11.27	6.18	2.91	20.36	57.45	1.82
Forest wellness	Absolutely	26	29	31	25	154	10
	Relatively	9.45	10.55	11.27	9.09	56.00	3.64

Source: Authors.

Table 3.
Results of the survey.

individuals in society. Moreover, this influence is crucial for the further interpretation of our results.

Based on the above, in further interpretation, we have examined the relationship between morbidity of individual respondents and the type of medicine, using the correlating coefficient examining linear dependence between two quantitative variables (**Table 4**).

We ascertain moderately high dependency between morbidity of individuals and their interest in medicine, mainly in conventional medicine (0.484698). This means that an individual, who is not ill, is not interested in influence of different types of medicine almost at all. However, we assume that the onset of illness is also associated with changes in the perception of different types of medicine. Because of the above and the correlations found, we are then able to abstract from indifferent attitudes and the resulting position of no influence on individual because of the ambiguous answers. Based on the results with such modification, we can conclude the conclusion related to the topic "Conventional versus complementary and alternative medicine from the viewpoint of perception of the public" as follows (**Figure 1**).

When it comes to mandatory types of medicine (must-be M), the individuals in case of illness definitely prefer conventional medicine due to the nonlinear and asymmetrical dependence between the importance and satisfaction of individuals with conventional and alternative medicine. These are the fundamental needs that people have in society; they are regarded as natural and automatic, and those who are sick either expect them or make them their top priority and first choice. We suppose that,

Monitored factor	Suffering from illness
Conventional medicine	0.484698
Regenerative environmental design	0.010944
Phytotherapy	0.082744
Aromatherapy	0.031775
Homeopathy	−0.067512
Flower therapy	−0.039081
Forest wellness	0.109966
Suffering from illness	−1
Disease-free	1

Table 4.
Correlation coefficients.

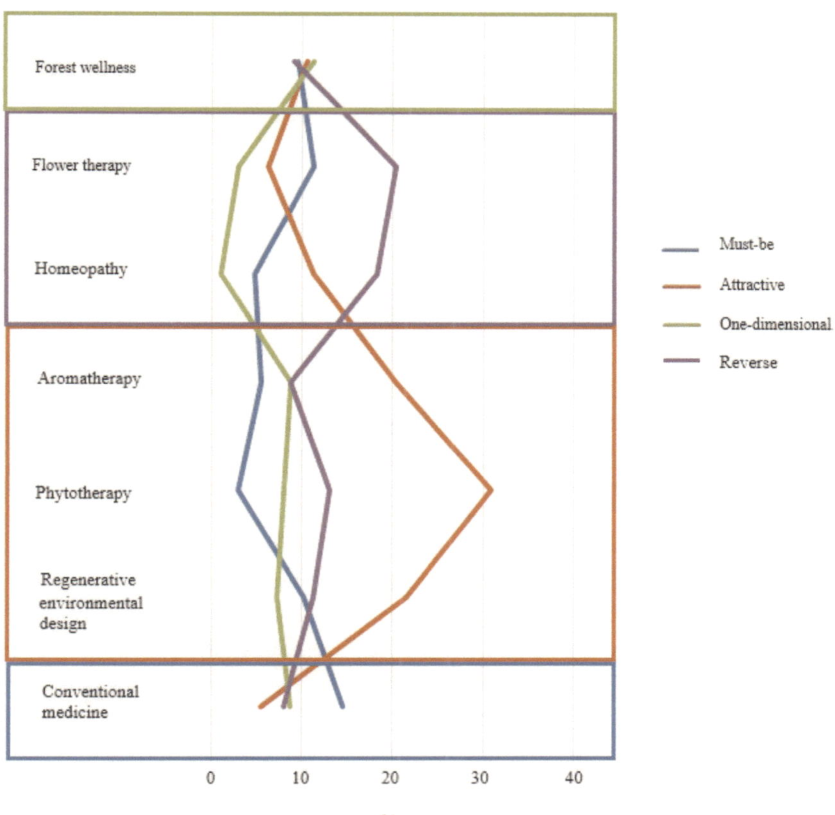

Figure 1.
The attitudes of the different types of medicine.

in case of illness, the individuals apply drugs or conventional therapy (over-the-counter drugs from the pharmacy, or those prescribed by a doctor), bed rest mode, and alternative therapy.

The most dominant is the group of attractive requirement of alternative medicine, which includes phytotherapy, regenerative environmental design, and aromatherapy. These types of medicine have a clear effect on satisfaction of individuals in case of their efficacy, as individuals do not expect these requirements (effects), and so, in case of their fulfillment, the individuals are satisfied; however, their ineffectiveness will not result in dissatisfaction of individuals.

In Slovakia, only forest wellness as anti-stress therapy is considered to be one-dimensional type of medicine by the society presented by individuals. The higher the rate of fulfillment of these requirements is, the more satisfied the individuals are, but these requirements are not automatically expected compared to mandatory requirements. This could be caused on by the fact that some people are unable to limit their personal or professional responsibilities when they are ill, and failing to fulfill these obligations raises stress levels.

Slovak society considers homeopathy and flower therapy to be reverse types of medicine according to the KANO classification. These forms of medicine reflect characteristics where people's responses are contradictory, which may indicate that they are unsure of the effectiveness of these alternative medicine treatments or that their effectiveness is only seen in certain conditions rather than for all kinds of illnesses.

The results indisputably demonstrate that conventional treatment is preferred over complementary or alternative medicine in Slovak society. In contrast to complementary and alternative medicine, which they find attractive, Slovaks' attitudes regarding conventional medicine are obligatory. According to the low correlation coefficient between the type of medicine and the morbidity of individual respondents, people who use alternative approaches to treatment of illnesses do so to lessen the symptoms associated with their illnesses or to lessen the side effects of conventional medicine. This also agrees with another studies result [17, 18, 47, 48].

Based on the aforementioned data, we can conclude that Slovak consumers are conventional consumers from a lifestyle perspective when considering the usage of conventional and alternative medicine. The type of segment behave as a very practical segment; the consumers do not have absolutely green attitudes but do have some "municipal" environmental behaviors such as recycling, energy conservation, and other similar behaviors. Cost savings drive this segment's behavior more than environmental consciousness. They mainly focus on sustainability benefits and economical, long-lasting, and reusable products. Prioritizing phytotherapy, regenerative environmental design, aromatherapy, and forest wellness over other types of alternative medicine is also based on Slovak traditions. Slovakia is one of the countries with the highest forest cover; the mountains cover 62% of Slovakia's territory and 49% of the population lives in them, placing the country in fourth place among the 25 states of the enlarged EU [49]. Herbs for phytotherapy and aromatherapy, forest for tourism, sports, anti-stress practices, forest wellness, and wood as a material for regenerative environmental design are easily available in Slovakia, which is why they have been used since time immemorial for alternative medicine, in construction and in other industries. While it may appear to us that the factors under investigation represent a contemporary trend, this is not entirely accurate; instead, they have their basis mainly in local customs and have been innovated with global cultures and trends. Today's alternative medicine, architecture, and leisure activities to relieve stress and increase human comfort follow traditions.

4. Conclusion

From a sociological perspective, it is interesting to watch how people in Slovakian society behave as consumers, particularly when it comes to how they view the many kinds of medicine that they look for, use, and expect will satisfy their needs considering the specificity of this economic sector. Regarding how Slovakian society views conventional versus complementary and alternative medicine, the market economy is currently seen as a specific kind of economic sector in which people behave like consumers with a focus on social and market economy principles.

Based on our findings, we can conclude that the Slovak lifestyle of consumers is conventional or potentially green. The Slovak consumer is a very practical segment that has environmental behavior such as recycling, energy-saving, and other similar behaviors. Rather, they focus on cost savings or the desire to waste less. They mainly focus on sustainability benefits and economical, long-lasting, and reusable products.

From the point of view of lifestyle and medicine based on the survey results, we can clearly state that conventional medicine is preferred to complementary and alternative medicine in Slovakia. The society in Slovakia perceives conventional medicine as a core medicine used in case of illness; it is the primary type of medicine seen as a natural and automatically used for diseases. Complementary and alternative medicine is also very interesting for the society in Slovakia, whereas it occupies a very attractive position. It is showing a clear effect on the satisfaction of individuals in society, in the case of action who did not expect. Complementary and alternative types of medicine are used more for the relief of symptoms associated with a disease, or elimination of the undesirable effects of conventional medicine.

Customer preferences of Slovak consumers from the point of view of lifestyle and of conventional, alternative medicine, architecture, and leisure activities to relieve stress and increase human comfort are rooted in traditions. Therefore, if we want to apply green practices and innovations in accordance with the lifestyle in Slovakia, it is necessary to measure the awareness of the issue and the benefits of sustainability, and the economic, long-term, and reusable benefits of the products and conduct targeted marketing campaigns (for example, environmental education activities, subsidy schemes for introducing ecological solutions, etc.).

Acknowledgements

This publication is the result of the project implementation: “Progressive research of performance properties of wood-based materials and products” (LignoPro), ITMS 313011 T720 supported by the Operational Programme Integrated Infrastructure (OPII) funded by the ERDF.

Conflict of interest

The authors declare no conflict of interest.

Notes

The chapter has 1.47 author sheet (AH), and it was created as part of the preparation of a future project "Business model of innovations based on the principle of sustainability".

Author details

Erika Loučanová* and Martina Nosáľová
Technical University in Zvolen, Zvolen, Slovakia

*Address all correspondence to: loucanova@tuzvo.sk

References

[1] Beery T, Stahl Olafsson A, Gentin S, Maurer M, Stålhammar S, Albert C, et al. Disconnection from nature: Expanding our understanding of human–nature relations. People and Nature. 2023;**5**: 470-488. DOI: 10.1002/pan3.10451

[2] Dong X, Shengmin L, Hongbo L, Zhi Y, Shichang L, Nianqi D. Love of nature as a mediator between connectedness to nature and sustainable consumption behavior. Journal of Cleaner Production. 2019;**42**:118451. DOI: 10.1016/j.jclepro.2019.118451

[3] Kautish P, Thaichon P, Soni P. Environmental values and sustainability: Mediating role of nature connectedness, and love for nature toward vegan food consumption. Journal of Consumer Behaviour. 2024;**23**(3): 1130-1145. DOI: 10.1002/cb.2267

[4] Velasco F, Cardenas M, Cardenas JJ, Martin SL. Key factors that influence consumer preferences for natural-hyped products. Psychology and Marketing. 2023;**40**:373-390. DOI: 10.1002/mar.21730

[5] Ogiemwonyi O, Alam MN, Alshareef R, Alsolamy M, Azizan NA, Mat N. Environmental factors affecting green purchase behaviors of the consumers: Mediating role of environmental attitude. Cleaner Environmental Systems. 2023;**10**: 100130. DOI: 10.1016/j.cesys.2023.100130

[6] Rahmah K, Satyaninggrat LMW. The effect of consumer characteristics and lifestyle toward purchase decision. Journal of Consumer Sciences. 2023; **8**(3):395-413. DOI: https://doi.org/10.29244/jcs.8.3.395-413

[7] United Nations. World Urbanization Prospects: The 2018 Revision; c2018. [Internet]. 2018. Available from: https://population.un.org/wup/publications/files/wup2018-keyfacts.pdf [Accessed: April 20, 2024]

[8] Mahato A, Ekka M. Nature within us: A sustainable lifestyle approach to connect with nature. International Journal of Advanced Biochemistry Research. 2023;**SP-7**:85-88. DOI: 10.33545/26174693.2023.v7.i2Sb.191

[9] WHO. Health and Environment in Sustainable Development: Five Years after the Earth Summit. 1997. Available from: https://iris.who.int/bitstream/handle/10665/63708/WHO_EHG_97.12_eng.pdf;jsessionid=1365E7808CC78BB37D94B32703224922?sequence=1 [Accessed: April 25, 2024]

[10] Martin L, White MP, Hunt A, Richardson M, Pahl S, Burt J. Nature contact, nature connectedness and associations with health, wellbeing and pro-environmental behaviours. Journal of Environmental Psychology. 2020;**68**: 101389. DOI: 10.1016/j.jenvp.2020.101389

[11] Sundermann M, Chielli D, Spell S. Nature as medicine: The 7th (unofficial) pillar of lifestyle medicine. American Journal of Lifestyle Medicine. 2023; **17**(5):717-729. DOI: 10.1177/15598276231174863

[12] Abookire SA, Ayala SG, Shadick NA. Supporting wellness, resilience, and community with forest therapy. Global Advances in Integrative Medicine and Health. 2024;**13**:1-7. DOI: 10.1177/27536130241246503

[13] King K, Church A. We don't enjoy nature like that': Youth identity and lifestyle in the countryside. Journal of

Rural Studies. 2013;**31**:67-76. DOI: doi.org/10.1016/j.jrurstud.2013.02.004

[14] Loučanová E, Nosáľová M. Social perceptions of conventional versus complementary and alternative medicine in Slovakia. Corvinus Journal of Sociology and Social Policy. 2020;**11**(2): 83-97. DOI: 10.14267/CJSSP.2020.2.5

[15] Zuraidah R, Hashima H, Yahya K, Mohamad S. Environmental conscious behaviour among male and female Malaysian consumers. OIDA International Journal of Sustainable Development. 2012;**4**(8):55-64

[16] Bodai BI, Nakata TE, Wong WT, et al. Lifestyle medicine: A brief review of its dramatic impact on health and survival. The Permanente Journal. 2018; **22**:17-025. DOI: 10.7812/TPP/17-025

[17] Astin JA, Harkness E, Ernst E. The efficacy of "distant healing": A systematic review of randomized trials. Annals of Internal Medicine. 2000; **132**(11):903-910. DOI: 10.7326/0003-4819-132-11-200006060-00009

[18] Astin JA. Why patients use alternative medicine: Results of a national study. Journal of the American Medical Association. 1998;**279**(19): 1548-1553. DOI: 10.1001/jama.279.19.1548

[19] Wemrell M, Merlo J, Mulinari S, Ch HA. Two-thirds of survey respondents in Southern Sweden used complementary or alternative medicine in 2015. Complementary Medicine Research. 2017;**24**(5):302-309. DOI: 10.1159/000464442

[20] NIH—National Institutes of Health. National Center for Complementary and Alternative Medicine (NCCAM): What Is Complementary and Alternative Medicine (CAM)? Publication No. D156. Bethesda: National Institutes of Health; 2006

[21] Purwono S, Nisa U, Astana PRW, Wijayaningsih RA, Wicaksono AJ, Wahyuningsih MSH, et al. Factors affecting the perception of Indonesian medical doctors on herbal medicine prescription in healthcare facilities: Qualitative and quantitative studies. Journal of Herbal Medicine. 2023;**42**: 100747. DOI: 10.1016/j.hermed.2023.100747

[22] Özkan O, Deniz T. An assessment of consumer demand for medicinal plants: A case of Istanbul. Eurasian Journal of Forest Science. 2023;**11**(1):1-13. DOI: 10.31195/ejejfs.1243329

[23] Robles AL, Chou S, Cole OJ, Hamid A, Griffiths A, Vedhara K. Psychological and social factors influencing patients' treatment selection for localised prostate cancer. In: Advances in Prostate Cancer. 2013. Available from: http://www.intechopen.com/books/advances-in-prostate-cancer/psychological-and-social-factors-influencing-patients-treatment-selection-for-localised-prostate-can [Accessed: April 25, 2024]

[24] Rabin LP. Psychiatric Aspects of End-Stage Renal Disease: Diagnosis and Management. New York: Academic Press; 1983

[25] Brown M, Dean S, Hay-Smith EJ, Taylor W, Baxter GD. Musculoskeletal pain and treatment choice: An exploration of illness perceptions and choices of conventional or complementary therapies. Disability and Rehabilitation. 2010;**32**:1645-1657. DOI: 10.3109/09638281003649896

[26] Porter MC, Diefenbach MA. Pushed and pulled: The role of affect and cognition in shaping CAM attitudes and

behavior among men treated for prostate cancer. Journal of Health Psychology. 2009;**14**:288-296. DOI: 10.1177/1359105308100

[27] Halama P, Gurňáková J. 2014: Need for structure and big five personality traits as predictors of decision making styles in health professionals. Studia Psychologica. 2014;**56**:171-180. DOI: 10.21909/sp.2014.03.658

[28] Kamhalová I, Halama P, Gurňáková J. Affect regulation and decision making in health-care professionals: Typology approach. Studia Psychologica. 2013;**55**:19-31. DOI: 10.21909/sp.2013.01.618

[29] Pilárik Ľ, Sarmány-Schuller I. Personality predictors of decision-making of medical rescuers. Studia Psychologica. 2011;**53**:175-184

[30] NMI—National Marketing Institute. LOHAS Segmentation Reflects Increasing Sophistication of Sustainability Marketplace. 2004. Available from: https://www.google.com/url?sa=t&source=web&rct=j&opi=89978449&url=https://faunalytics.org/wp-content/uploads/2015/05/Citation887.pdf&ved=2ahUKEwj56rfH2YeHAxWb_rsIHc9QCDMQFnoECBwQAQ&usg=AOvVaw29kcXDS5YUohuncQYK7ZQq/ [Accessed: December 20, 2023]

[31] Ottman J. A Smart New Way to Segment Green Consumers. 2024. Available from: http://www.greenmarketing.com/blog/comments/a-smart-new-way-to-segment-green-consumers/ [Accessed: February 2, 2024]

[32] Ziaei-Bideh A, Namakshenas-Jahromi M. Profiling Green Consumers with Data Mining. London: IntechOpen; 2020, 2020. DOI: 10.5772/intechopen.83373

[33] Conway P. Stromy, ktoré léčí. Praha: TRITON; 2001. 373p

[34] Braun L. Herbal medicines and interactions with conventional medicines used to manage diabetes. In: Dunning T, editor. Complementary Therapies and the Management of Diabetes and Vascular Disease: A Matter of Balance. Marrickville, Australia: Elsevier, John Wiley and Sons; 2006. p. 211. 2007. Available from: https://en.wikipedia.org/wiki/Phytotherapy#cite_note-Dunning2007-1 [Accessed: February 25, 2024]

[35] Aromatherapy. Better Health Channel. 2024. Available from: https://en.wikipedia.org/wiki/Aromatherapy#cite_note-1 [Accessed: April 20, 2024]

[36] Hahnemann S. The Homœopathic Medical Doctrine or "Organon of the Healing Art". Dublin: W.F. Wakeman; 1833. Available from: https://en.wikipedia.org/wiki/Homeopathy#cite_note-Hahnemann-1. pp. 48-49 [Accessed: February 25, 2024]

[37] Vohra DS. Bach Flower Remedies: A Comprehensive Study. New Delhi: Health Harmony; 2002. 258 p

[38] Gibbons LV. Regenerative—The new sustainable? Sustainability. 2020; **12**(13):5483

[39] Nigudkar S. Regenerative Sustainable Design. 2024. Available from: https://www.re-thinkingthefuture.com/sustainable-architecture/a6024-regenerative-sustainable-design/ [Accessed: June 25, 2024]

[40] Mihardja EJ, Alisjahbana S, Agustini PM, Sari DAP, Pardede TS.

Forest wellness tourism destination branding for supporting disaster mitigation: A case of batur UNESCO global geopark, Bali. International Journal of Geoheritage and Parks. 2023; **11**(1):169-181. DOI: 10.1016/j.ijgeop.2023.01.003

[41] Chen HR, Cheng BW. A case study in solving customer complaints based on the 8Ds method and Kano model. Journal of Chinese Institute of Industrial Engineers. 2010;**5**:339-350. DOI: 10.1080/10170669.2010.495508

[42] Chen LS, Liu CH, Ch HC, Lin Ch SC. Kano model: A novel approach for discovering attractive quality elements. Total Quality Management. 2010;**21**: 1189-1214. DOI: 10.1080/14783363.2010.529347

[43] Sharif Ullah AMM, Tamaki J. Analysis of Kano-model-based customer needs for product development. Systems Engineering. 2011;**4**:154-172. DOI: 10.1002/sys.20168

[44] Cohen J, Cohen P, West SG, Aiken LS. Applied Multiple Regression/Correlation Analysis for the Behavioral Sciences. 3rd ed. New York: Routledge; 2013. 536 p. DOI: 10.4324/9780203774441

[45] Tontini G, Solberg Søilen K, Silveira A. How do interactions of Kano model attributes affect customer satisfaction? An analysis based on psychological foundations. Total Quality Management and Business Excellence. 2013;**24**:1253-1271. DOI: 10.1080/14783363.2013.836790

[46] Statistical Office of the Slovak Republic. 2023. Available from: https://slovak.statistics.sk/ [Accessed: March 20, 2024]

[47] McCaffrey AM, Pugh GF, O'Connor BB. Understanding patient preference for integrative medical care: Results from patient focus groups. Journal of General Internal Medicine. 2007;**22**:1500-1505

[48] Lo CB, Desmond RA, Meleth S. Inclusion of complementary and alternative medicine in US state comprehensive cancer control plans: Baseline data. Journal of Cancer Education. 2009;**24**:249-253. DOI: 10.1080/08858190902972897

[49] Sermek R. Slovensko jednou z najhornatejších krajín EÚ. 2024. Available from: https://svet.sme.sk/c/1309858/slovensko-jednou-z-najhornatejsich-krajin-eu.html [Accessed: June 20, 2024]

Section 3

Aromatherapy

Chapter 5

Aromatherapy: Historical, Phytochemical Insights, and Therapeutic Applications

Chadi Khatib

Abstract

This chapter delves into the holistic practice of aromatherapy, which harnesses the therapeutic potential of aromatic compounds in essential oils derived from medicinal plants to support physical, emotional, and mental health. The chapter traces the historical roots of aromatherapy, emphasizing its revered role in ancient civilizations, where aromatic substances were utilized for their healing properties. Examining aromatherapy through chemical, biochemical, and pharmacological lenses underscores the diverse therapeutic applications of essential oils. A focal point of the chapter is the introduction of the aroma wheel, a tool that categorizes and elucidates the intricate scents of essential oils, aiding in their practical application. The chapter also explores the extensive trade of spices and aromatic substances—such as musk, ambergris, camphor, and sandalwood—during the medieval period, particularly in the East and Spain. A notable figure in this historical narrative is the Spanish physician and aromatherapist Albucasis, who extensively addressed the use of aromatherapy in the nineteenth book of his influential work, *Kitab al-Tasrif*. By offering a comprehensive overview of the historical, chemical, and therapeutic dimensions of aromatherapy, this chapter serves as a valuable resource for researchers and practitioners in natural medicine, illustrating how the power of scent can significantly enhance health and well-being.

Keywords: aromatherapy, medicinal plants, essential oils, phytochemicals, therapeutic properties, aromatic compounds, biochemical pathways, pharmacological effects, holistic healing

1. Introduction

Aromatherapy, the practice of using aromatic plant extracts to promote physical, emotional, and spiritual well-being, boasts a rich history across various cultures [1]. Ancient civilizations in India, China, Egypt, and Greece recognized the profound effects of aromatic plants, essential oils, and perfumes on health and spirituality [2–4]. For example, perfumes were integral to treatments and rituals in Pharaonic, Greek, and Roman societies [5]. The Arabic terms "El-tib" or "Tyyb" and "Itr" or "Ottor" refer to fragrant substances used for enhancing aromas or treating illnesses, encompassing both animal and botanical elements such as musk, ambergris, cloves, camphor, sandalwood, and aloeswood [6]. The term "aromatherapy," coined in the early twentieth century by René-Maurice Gattefossé, refers to the use of essential oils through various methods, including massage, baths, and inhalation [7]. The related field of "aromachology" studies the physiological effects of scents [8]. Today, aromatherapy is gaining renewed interest as a complementary therapy, with research focusing on how essential oils interact with the body and mind to reveal their therapeutic potential [9]. The historical trade of perfumes and aromatic plants has evolved into a vibrant field of study, expanding our understanding of their holistic health benefits [10, 11].

2. Historical perspectives of aromatherapy

2.1 Origin of aromatherapy

The origins of aromatherapy can be traced back to ancient Babylon (circa 2000–1000 BC), where aromatic plants and spices were traded along early routes in South and Central Asia [12–14]. Ancient Egyptians pioneered the use of aromatic oils for medical, cosmetic, and religious purposes, as evidenced by inscriptions in temples, such as Deir el-Bahari, Philae, and Edfu [15]. Cleopatra's use of jasmine oil to captivate Mark Antony underscores the cultural significance of aromatics [16, 17]. Egyptians developed advanced methods for extracting essential oils, such as chamomile, which were used in therapeutic treatments and mummification, reflecting their knowledge of preservation and medicinal qualities [18].

In China, aromatics were primarily used in incense, an early form of aromatherapy, to cleanse spaces and promote health, integrated into traditional medicine and spiritual practices [19]. Ayurveda in India extensively utilized aromatherapy, with substances like saffron and milk plasters employed for their medicinal and aromatic properties. For example, these materials were used to purify air during the construction of the Temple of Minerva [20, 21].

Romans incorporated aromatic oils into daily routines, such as bathing, to promote relaxation and enhance sensory experiences, highlighting their appreciation for luxury and well-being [22, 23]. The amalgamation of Greek, Arabic, and Islamic traditions significantly advanced aromatherapy. Greek scholars like Hippocrates and Dioscorides documented the medicinal uses of aromatic plants, a knowledge preserved and expanded during the Islamic Golden Age. Arab merchants from the Quraysh tribe were instrumental in spreading perfumes throughout the Middle East [24–27]. Innovations in extraction techniques such as steam distillation were advanced by Islamic scholars like Jābir ibn Hayyān (Geber) and Al-Kindi (Alkindus), with figures like Avicenna (Ibn Sina) refining floral oil distillation. Abū al-Qāsim al-Zahrawī (Albucasis) detailed distillation methods in his seminal work, *Kitab al-Tasrif*, which includes insights into perfume preparation and therapeutic applications [28–30].

2.2 Modalities of aromatherapy in traditional systems

Traditional systems utilize a range of methods to harness the therapeutic benefits of essential oils and aromatic plants [31]. Ayurveda employs oils like sandalwood and jasmine through massage, steam inhalation, and baths to balance doshas [32].

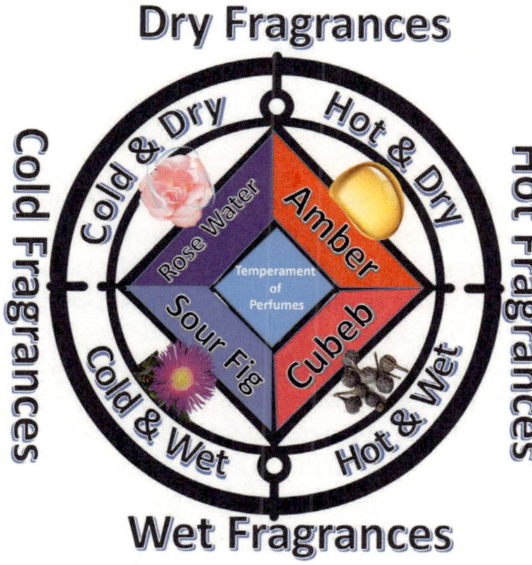

Figure 1.
Temperament of perfumes.

Traditional Chinese Medicine (TCM) uses aromatics like camphor and ginger to harmonize Qi, often in combination with acupuncture and herbal treatments [33].

Unani medicine, rooted in Greek humoral theory, classifies substances based on their qualities and therapeutic effects. Albucasis categorized perfumes into types based on their temperament: hot and dry (amber, nutmeg), cold and wet (sour fig, lichen), cold and dry (rose water, camphor), and hot and wet (cubeb) (**Figure 1**) [6]. He described external methods like sitz baths, steam inhalation, incense, and perfumed ornaments; topical methods including aromatic oils, massage agents, and aromatic detergents; and internal methods such as snuff and aromatic water [6]. Fragrances were tailored by gender, age, and season, highlighting a sophisticated understanding of scent effects on well-being [6]. In our days, the Saudi Arabian perfume company Abdul Samad Al Qurashi is considered one of the notable perfume companies that have developed the concept of Arabic perfume and its various forms, relying on the rich Arab heritage in the production and creation of fragrances [34].

The circle represents the four moods of scents in Unani medicine: hot, cold, dry, and wet. Each mood is associated with specific scents: hot and dry (amber), cold and wet (sour fig), cold and dry (rose water), and hot and wet (cubeb). This figure is an original design by the author, inspired by interpretations of ancient manuscripts by Albucasis.

The classification of perfumes based on the temperament in Unani medicine (UM) aligns with the humoral theory. Each category reflects the qualities of the perfumes and their potential therapeutic effects.

3. Phytochemical insights of aromatherapy

3.1 Chemical structures

Understanding the chemical structures of essential oils is crucial for their therapeutic applications. Essential oils are concentrated plant extracts consisting of primary compounds for therapeutic effects and supplementary compounds that enhance scent and efficacy.

3.1.1 Main compounds

Essential or volatile oils are concentrated extracts from plants that capture their aromatic properties and are composed of various chemical groups, each contributing distinct scents and therapeutic effects. The primary constituents are terpenoids, which include monoterpenes and sesquiterpenes. Monoterpenes, such as limonene, pinene, and myrcene, are known for their uplifting and decongestant effects, providing fresh, bright citrus notes and are commonly found in citrus oils and coniferous plants. Sesquiterpenes, like caryophyllene, farnesene, and bisabolol, are heavier molecules that contribute to earthy scents and are recognized for their anti-inflammatory and analgesic properties. They are typically found in oils like chamomile and sandalwood [35–38].

Other significant compounds include aromatic esters, aldehydes, ketones, and phenylpropanoids. Aromatic esters, such as linalyl acetate, benzyl acetate, and ethyl butyrate, are appreciated for their sweet, fruity aromas, and calming effects, commonly used in perfumes and found in oils like lavender and ylang-ylang. Aldehydes and ketones, including citral, vanillin, and cinnamaldehyde, are valued for their fresh, citrusy, or sweet notes, contributing pleasant aromas and antimicrobial properties to both natural and synthetic perfumery. Phenylpropanoids, such as eugenol, cinnamaldehyde, and anethole, impart spicy notes and are known for their antimicrobial and antioxidant properties, with eugenol in clove oil being notable for its pain-relieving effects (**Figure 2**) [39–41].

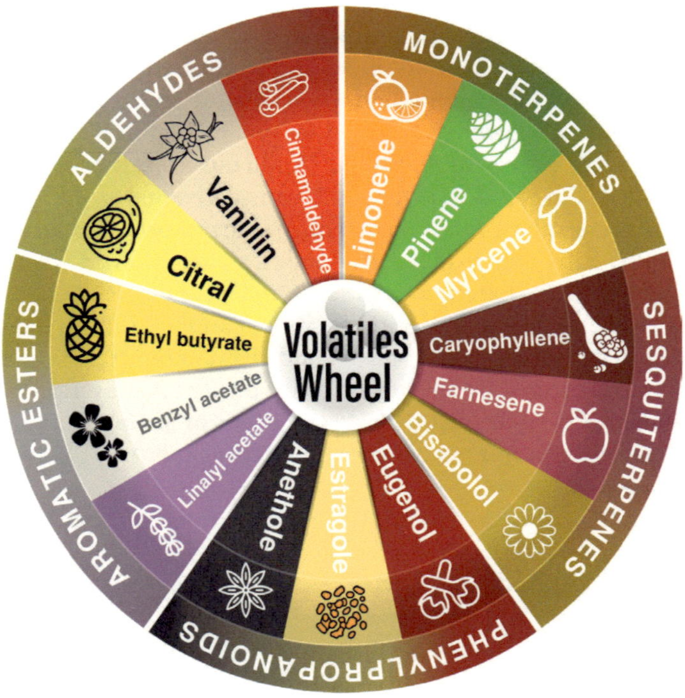

Figure 2.
Volatiles wheel.

This original infographic design by the author represents the five major groups of chemical compounds found in essential oils: monoterpenes (e.g., limonene, pinene, and myrcene), sesquiterpenes (e.g., caryophyllene, farnesene, and bisabolol), phenylpropanoids (e.g., eugenol, cinnamaldehyde, and anethole), aromatic esters (e.g., linalyl acetate, benzyl acetate, and ethyl butyrate), and aldehydes and ketones (e.g., citral, vanillin, and cinnamaldehyde). Each group is illustrated with vector representations of these example compounds.

The Volatiles Wheel showcases the diversity of chemical compounds that contribute to the aromatic profiles of essential oils. Monoterpenes and sesquiterpenes form the backbone of these profiles, imparting citrus and earthy notes, respectively. Phenylpropanoids add spiciness, while aromatic esters and aldehydes/ketones contribute floral and sweet aromas. This figure, is inspired by the chemical composition of volatile oils.

The diversity of these compounds not only defines the aromatic profile of essential oils but also influences their therapeutic properties, which are shaped by factors like extraction methods and cultivation conditions [42].

Animal-derived scents and synthetic fragrances also contribute to the complexity of aromatherapy. Animal-derived scents include hydrocarbons, alcohols, and esters, while synthetic fragrances are categorized by chemical structures, such as hydrocarbons, alcohols, esters, and aldehydes [43–45].

3.1.2 Complementary compounds

Complementary compounds enhance the efficacy and safety of aromatherapy products. Carrier oils like jojoba and sweet almond oil dilute essential oils for safe topical use and aid in skin absorption [46, 47]. Waxes such as beeswax provide structural integrity to candles [48]. Emulsifiers and surfactants stabilize emulsions in lotions and creams [49]. Ethanol dissolves aromatic compounds in perfumes, facilitating their release [50]. Fixatives like terpenoid-rich resins extend the longevity of scents [51]. Propellants in deodorants enable fine spray applications [52]. While charcoal and binders are used in incense [53, 54]. Understanding the chemical structures of these compounds is essential for their effective use in aromatherapy and perfumery.

3.2 Analytical techniques

3.2.1 Chemical analysis techniques

Essential oils can be analyzed using several techniques. Gas chromatography (GC) separates and analyzes volatile compounds [55]. Mass spectrometry (MS) identifies molecular weight and structure [56]. Optical rotation (OR) measures the angle of polarized light to assess purity [57]. The refractive index (RI) evaluates light refraction to determine oil quality [58]. Specific gravity (SG) is used to verify authenticity and concentration [59]. Finally, structure–activity relationships (SAR) analyze the chemical structure and biological activity of the compounds [60].

3.2.2 Techniques for assessing fragrances

Various methods are used to evaluate fragrances. The Perfumery Radar (PR) methodology categorizes perfumes into olfactory families [61]. Sensory experiments include techniques such as intensity ranking, semantic profiling, and panel testing [62–64]. Gustatory smell correlation studies examine the relationship between aroma and taste, emphasizing how the sense of smell influences taste perception [65]. Additionally, the electronic nose system replicates the human olfactory system for rapid and objective odor analysis [66].

3.3 Categorization of aromatherapy ingredients

Fragrances in aromatherapy are categorized based on their scent profiles, which are closely linked to their chemical structures. For example, citrus scents like limonene, floral scents like jasmone, aldehyde scents like octanal, and oriental scents like vanillin are categorized this way. Other examples include fruity scents like isoamyl acetate, fougère scents like coumarin, watery (marine) scents like calone, conifer scents like alpha-pinene, chypre scents like labdane, herbaceous scents like eucalyptol, green scents like cis-3-hexenal, spicy scents like cinnamaldehyde, woody scents like santalol, fresh scents like cis-3-hexenol, aromatic scents like linalool, musk scents like muscone, animal-like scents like civetone, and vegetable-like scents like hexanal (**Figure 3**) [67].

This figure presents the chemical structures of key fragrance compounds found in aromatherapy, organized by their scent profiles. Examples include citrus (limonene), floral (jasmone), aldehyde (octanal), and oriental (vanillin) scents. The figure also includes other scent profiles, such as fruity (isoamyl acetate), fougère (coumarin), watery/marine (calone), conifer (alpha-pinene), chypre (labdane), herbaceous (eucalyptol), green (cis-3-hexenal), spicy (cinnamaldehyde), woody (santalol), fresh (cis-3-hexenol), aromatic (linalool), musk (muscone), animal-like (civetone), and vegetable-like (hexanal). Each scent profile is illustrated with its corresponding chemical structure to highlight the relationship between molecular composition and fragrance characteristics.

The figure expands on the traditional aroma wheel by categorizing 18 distinct scent profiles in aromatherapy, each represented by a specific chemical compound. This organization emphasizes the direct link between the chemical structure of a compound and its associated scent profile, demonstrating how the molecular makeup of a fragrance ingredient determines its aromatic properties.

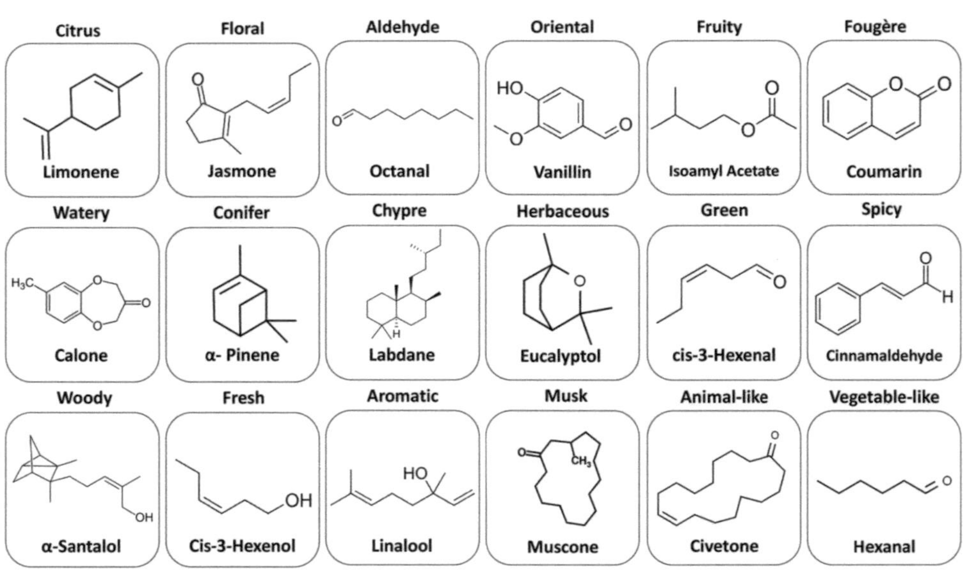

Figure 3.
Chemical structures of notable aromatherapy fragrance compounds.

The categorization of aromatherapy ingredients extends beyond chemical structures to include organized scent families, as depicted in the fragrance wheel (FW). This wheel groups scents into families such as floral, oriental, woody, fresh, and aromatic. For instance, the floral family encompasses subgroups like floral, soft floral, and floral oriental, featuring scents such as jasmine and rose water, characterized by fresh-cut flowers, aldehydes, powdery notes, and sweet spices. The oriental family includes soft oriental, oriental, and woody oriental subgroups, with scents like ambergris, noted for incense, amber, and oriental resins. The woody family comprises woods, mossy woods, dry woods, and aromatic woods, with examples like frankincense and sandalwood, characterized by dry woods, leather, oakmoss, and vetiver. The fresh family includes citrus, fruity, green, and water subgroups, with scents such as lavender and sweet orange, characterized by aquatic notes, green notes, fruits, and citrus oils. The aromatic family features scents like rose water [68, 69].

Uniquely, the fougère family is positioned at the center of the fragrance wheel, combining elements from all four other families, which gives it universal appeal. Oak moss is a classic example of a fougère scent [68, 69]. Fragrances are also structured within a pyramid, where top notes represent the initial light scents, middle notes provide the core character, and base notes offer long-lasting depth [70]. Additionally, perfumes are classified by concentration levels, ranging from the intense Parfum (Extrait) to the lighter Eau Fraîche [71].

Synthetic aroma chemicals, integral to modern perfumery, are divided into three categories: commodities, which are basic and widely used; specialties, which are unique ingredients for distinct fragrances; and captives, proprietary compounds exclusive to certain fragrance houses [72]. To support the categorization and understanding of these fragrances, various databases and tools, including the Modified Hexagon (MH), H&R Catalog (H&R), Fragrantica (FR), and Osmoz (OZ), are utilized [73, 74]. Furthermore, major fragrance houses like Firmenich and Givaudan contribute significantly to the industry with their extensive research databases [75].

4. Therapeutic applications of fragrance substances

Aromatherapy employs fragrance compounds, such as essential oils, for therapeutic purposes; these oils can be inhaled or applied topically to influence the limbic system, which is responsible for emotions, memories, and physiological responses [76]. This review will categorize these oils based on their therapeutic applications and their pharmaceutical, nutraceutical, and cosmeceutical forms.

4.1 Physical health

Essential oils provide numerous benefits for physical health, including:

- *Respiratory health*: Eucalyptus and peppermint oils alleviate symptoms of colds and respiratory infections [77].

- *Digestive health*: Ginger and fennel oils support digestion and relieve nausea [78].

- *Pain relief*: Lavender and chamomile oils possess analgesic properties for pain management [79, 80].

- *Immune system support*: Tea tree, eucalyptus, and thyme oils enhance the body's natural defenses [81].
- *Antibacterial properties*: Certain essential oils, such as tea tree, oregano, and thyme, exhibit antibacterial activity against various pathogens [82].
- *Antiviral activity*: Oils like peppermint, lemongrass, and cinnamon may help fight viral infections [83].
- *Antifungal properties*: Clove, lavender, and peppermint oils are effective against fungal infections [84].
- *Cytotoxic and anticancer properties*: Essential oils like thyme, lemongrass, and ginger have shown cytotoxic effects on cancer cells [85, 86]. These oils may exert anticancer effects through several mechanisms, including the induction of apoptosis by triggering programmed cell death in cancer cells, cell cycle arrest by halting cancer cell proliferation, inhibition of angiogenesis by blocking the formation of new blood vessels needed for tumor growth, and modulation of signaling pathways involved in cancer progression [87–90].

4.2 Emotional and psychological well-being

Aromatherapy is widely recognized for its emotional and psychological benefits [91].

- *Reducing stress*: Lavender and bergamot oils are known for their calming effects [92, 93].
- *Enhancing mood*: Citrus oils like orange and lemon uplift and energize [94].
- *Improving seep*: Oils such as valerian and sandalwood promote restful sleep [95].
- *Spiritual and holistic benefits*: Many cultures utilize aromatherapy for spiritual and holistic healing, using essential oils like frankincense and myrrh in rituals to enhance meditation and spiritual practices [96]. Aromatherapy is also incorporated into holistic health practices to balance the body, mind, and spirit. Drawing on techniques from various traditional medicine systems and often being used in spa and massage therapy as complementary treatments, this integrative approach supports skin health, detoxification, and emotional balance [97–101].

4.3 Skin and beauty

Essential oils significantly contribute to skin care [102, 103].

- *Antiaging*: Oils like rose and frankincense help reduce signs of aging [104].
- *Acne treatment*: Tea tree oil is effective for managing acne [105].
- *Moisturizing*: Oils such as jojoba and almonds with aromatic oils provide hydration [106].

- *Hair care*: Essential oils stimulate hair follicles and promote growth, such as rosemary oil, lavender oil, and peppermint oil [107–109]. Additionally, essential oils can help maintain a healthy scalp by addressing dandruff and irritation, such as tea tree oil and cedarwood oil [110, 111].

4.4 Pharmaceutical forms of aromatherapy

- *Internal*: Essential oils are incorporated into products like herbal teas [112] and aromatic beverages, including those made with oregano and thyme [113]. Capsules such as Rowatinex® (Rx) contain essential oils like α-pinene, β-pinene, camphene, borneol, anethol, fenchone, cineole, and olive oil, which are used internally to promote urinary health [114]. Additionally, essential oils serve as functional foods and dietary supplements [115]. Their application as natural additives for extending the shelf life of food products has also gained significant attention [116].

- *Topical*: Essential oils find extensive use in topical applications such as massage oils [117]; lotions, creams, and other cosmetic preparations [118]; and balms and salves [100]. They are also integrated into bath oils and salts [119, 120], as well as shampoos and conditioners [121]. Additionally, hydrosols—commonly known as floral waters—are applied directly to the skin, offering a variety of benefits [122].

- *External*: Essential oils are externally applied in various ways, including through diffusers and sprays to disperse scents into the air [123–125], as well as in inhalation products that offer respiratory relief [126, 127]. They are also used in aromatic candles and incense to create a calming atmosphere [128, 129]. Natural perfumes provide both aromatic and therapeutic benefits [130–132]. Additionally, essential oils are incorporated into household cleaning products and linen sprays, which offer antiseptic properties and refreshing scents, promoting a healthier living environment [133, 134].

5. Safety considerations in aromatherapy

5.1 Toxicity and contraindications

Essential oils should be used with caution to avoid adverse effects. Dilute them to 1–5% in a carrier oil to prevent skin irritation [135], and perform a patch test to check for allergies or irritation [136, 137]. Consult a professional before using essential oils during pregnancy or on children due to potential risks [135]. Avoid sun exposure for 12 hours after applying photosensitive oils like bergamot, lemon, and lime [138]. Ingestion should only occur under the guidance of a healthcare professional, as essential oils can be toxic if swallowed [139].

5.2 Interactions with medicines

Essential oils can interact with various medications, potentially altering their effectiveness or increasing side effects [140], such as enhancing bleeding risk with blood thinners [141], causing serotonin syndrome with antidepressants, affecting blood sugar levels with diabetes medications, counteracting antihypertensives, and increasing sedation with sedatives [142], so consultation with a healthcare provider is essential.

5.3 Regulatory guidelines

These guidelines include the International Fragrance Association (IFRA), which sets safety standards for fragrance ingredients in consumer products [143], and the Cosmetic Ingredient Review (CIR), which assesses the safety of cosmetic ingredients, including fragrances [144].

6. Future directions and innovations in aromatherapy and fragrance industries

The aromatherapy and fragrance industries are undergoing significant evolution driven by technological innovations, expanded therapeutic applications, and integration with modern medicine.

6.1 Technological advancements

Innovations in biotechnology are enabling sustainable fragrance production, including creating unique, non-natural aromas [145]. Advanced extraction and analytical techniques, such as chromatography and nuclear magnetic resonance spectroscopy (NMR), are improving the precision and efficacy of essential oils in therapeutic uses [146, 147]. Additionally, sophisticated delivery systems like microencapsulation and nanoemulsions are enhancing the stability and longevity of aromatherapy products, leading to the development of solid fragrances and gels [148].

6.2 Expanded applications

Research is extending aromatherapy's role in managing chronic conditions, mental health issues, and cognitive enhancement. For example, lavender oil is studied for its calming effects, while peppermint oil is used for cognitive stimulation and headache relief [149]. The trend toward functional fragrances, which offer mood enhancement and stress relief, is also gaining traction as consumers seek products that support overall well-being [150].

6.3 Integration with modern medicine

Aromatherapy is increasingly integrated into conventional medicine, with healthcare professionals using essential oils in clinical settings to improve patient care. Lavender and peppermint oils are commonly used for their anxiolytic and anti-nausea properties, respectively [31]. Essential oils are also employed in complementary therapies alongside conventional treatments in areas like palliative care and mental health support [151].

6.4 Advanced delivery systems

New delivery systems are enhancing the user experience of aromatherapy products. Microencapsulation ensures long-lasting fragrance release, used in scented textiles and personal care items [152, 153]. Nanoemulsions improve the stability and penetration of essential oils in skin care and aromatherapy [154, 155]. Solid fragrances and gels offer portability and convenience [156, 157].

6.5 Personalized fragrances and consumer trends

The rise of artificial intelligence (AI) and genetic testing is enabling the creation of personalized fragrances tailored to individual preferences and body chemistries [158, 159]. Additionally, there is increasing demand for sustainable, eco-friendly practices in the industry, with companies adopting ethical sourcing and eco-friendly packaging to meet consumer expectations [160].

6.6 Digital and interactive fragrance experiences

The digitalization of fragrance experiences is an emerging trend, with virtual reality (VR) and augmented reality (AR) technologies creating immersive scent explorations in virtual environments [161, 162]. Digital scent technologies, though still experimental, hold potential for future applications in digital media and entertainment [163].

7. Conclusion

Aromatherapy exemplifies the integration of ancient wisdom with modern scientific advancements to foster holistic health and wellness. This practice, rooted in the rituals and medicinal uses of aromatic substances by ancient civilizations, has evolved into a sophisticated therapeutic modality. The historical contributions of figures such as Albucasis have left an indelible mark on contemporary practices, especially within the perfume industry, bridging traditional knowledge with current therapeutic methodologies.

Today, aromatherapy is widely recognized as a comprehensive practice within complementary, alternative, and traditional medicine (CAM/TM). It encompasses a diverse range of techniques, including perfume therapy, functional fragrances, and scent therapy. These methods leverage essential oils and other fragrant substances across pharmaceutical, cosmeceutical, and nutraceutical domains, as well as environmental applications. The growing body of research underscores the potential of aromatherapy as a complementary approach to holistic health, demonstrating its efficacy in enhancing patient experiences and outcomes.

The extensive range of fragrance compounds—both natural and synthetic—plays a pivotal role in tailoring treatments to address specific therapeutic or sensory needs. This versatility extends beyond perfumery to encompass skincare, beauty, and overall well-being. Understanding and utilizing the full spectrum of aromatic substances is crucial for optimizing their therapeutic benefits.

Recent trends highlight not only the sensory pleasure derived from fragrances but also their significant therapeutic effects. Scents influence the central nervous system through the limbic system, affecting relaxation, mood, and overall well-being. This interaction suggests that incorporating pleasant fragrances into daily routines can offer substantial improvements in mental and emotional health.

Looking ahead, ongoing research and technological innovations are expected to unveil new applications for aromatherapy and enhance our understanding of the therapeutic properties of scents. Advances in "perfume engineering," integrating chemistry, neuroscience, and psychology, are advancing our knowledge of how fragrance compounds impact human perception and well-being. This interdisciplinary approach is paving the way for more precise and effective aromatic therapies.

Sustainability presents both challenges and opportunities in the field. Responsible harvesting of aromatic plants is crucial, particularly as demand for eco-friendly products increases. Essential oils are emerging as promising alternatives to harmful chemicals used in pesticides, preservatives, and cleaning agents. Additionally, the growing concern over bacterial resistance highlights the potential of natural compounds like essential oils to complement traditional antibiotics in combating pathogens.

Future research should explore the classification of essential oils based on their temperamental qualities, such as cooling versus warming properties. Understanding how oils with opposing characteristics interact could lead to innovative therapeutic applications and enhance the efficacy of aromatherapy.

In conclusion, the future of aromatherapy is promising, marked by technological advancements, expanded therapeutic applications, and greater integration with modern medicine. The increasing recognition of therapeutic fragrances and the evolving field of fragrance therapy reflect a growing acknowledgment of the benefits of essential oils for holistic health. With strong consumer interest, technological progress, and deeper connections with healthcare, the aromatherapy and fragrance industries are poised for significant growth and a dynamic future, reflecting the continuous evolution of this ancient practice into a modern therapeutic tool.

Acknowledgements

I would like to express my sincere gratitude to Al-Manara University and its dedicated administrative and academic staff. My special thanks go to Dr. Safwan Al-Asaf, President of the University; Dr. Muthanna Al-Qubaili, Secretary of the University; and Dr. Kinda Darwish, Dean of the Faculty of Pharmacy. I also extend my appreciation to the remarkable Ms. Faten Al-Ali for her support.

Additionally, I am deeply grateful to the Board of Directors of the Syrian Scientific Society for Herbal Medicine, Complementary Medicine, Homeopathy, and Nutrition for their ongoing scientific support and valuable contributions.

Additional information

- The author acknowledges the use of ChatGPT for language polishing of the manuscript.

- The author created all figures presented in this manuscript.

Acronyms and abbreviations

TCM	Traditional Chinese Medicine
UM	Unani medicine
IFRA	International Fragrance Association
CIR	Cosmetic Ingredient Review
GC	gas chromatography

DOI: http://dx.doi.org/10.5772/intechopen.1006954

MS	mass spectrometry
OR	optical rotation
RI	refractive index
SG	specific gravity
SAR	structure–activity relationships
PR	Perfumery Radar
NMR	nuclear magnetic resonance spectroscopy
FW	fragrance wheel
MH	Modified Hexagon
H&R	H&R Catalog
FR	Fragrantica
OZ	Osmoz
Rx	Rowatinex®
CAM/TM	complementary, alternative, and traditional medicine

Author details

Chadi Khatib
Manara University, Latakia, Syria

*Address all correspondence to: chadi.khatib@gmail.com

References

[1] Dwivedi A, Mishra R, Chaturved M. Aromatherapy a holistic cure: Current approaches and future concerns. International Journal of Pharmaceutical and Life Sciences. 2010;**1**(1):23-29

[2] Giannenas I et al. The history of herbs, medicinal and aromatic plants, and their extracts: Past, current situation and future perspectives. In: Feed Additives. Cambridge, Massachusetts: Academic Press; 2020. pp. 1-18. DOI: 10.1016/b978-0-12-814700-9.00001-7

[3] Halcón LL, Buckle J. Aromatherapy. In: Complementary and Alternative Therapies in Nursing. 7th ed. New York: Springer; 2014. p. 323. DOI: 10.1891/9780826196347.0020

[4] Farrar AJ, Farrar FC. Clinical aromatherapy. Nursing Clinics. 2020;**55**(4):489-504. DOI: 10.1016/j.cnur.2020.06.015

[5] Vatca A, Vatca S. The history and use of perfume in human civilization. Agricultura. 2017;**103**:3-4

[6] Alraghran A, Khatib C. The new informations about aromatherapy and scents edited by Albucasis. Journal of the International Society for the History of Islamic Medicine. 2015;**14**:64-83

[7] Thangaleela S et al. Essential oils, phytoncides, aromachology, and aromatherapy—A review. Applied Sciences. 2022;**12**(9):4495. DOI: 10.3390/app12094495

[8] Herz RS. Aromatherapy facts and fictions: A scientific analysis of olfactory effects on mood, physiology and behavior. International Journal of Neuroscience. 2009;**119**(2):263-290. DOI: 10.1080/00207450802333953

[9] Farrer-Halls G. The spirit in aromatherapy: Working with intuition. Singing Dragon. 2014:41-44

[10] Maiti S, Geetha KA. Medicinal and Aromatic Plants in India. 2008.

[11] Inoue M, Hayashi S, Craker LE. Role of medicinal and aromatic plants: Past, present, and future. Pharmacognosy-Medicinal Plants. 2019;**13**:1. DOI: 10.5772/intechopen.82497

[12] Rimmel E. The Book of Perfumes. London: Chapman and Hall; 1867

[13] Balasubramanian N. Scented oils and perfumes. In: Chemical Technology in Antiquity. Washington: American Chemical Society; 2015. pp. 219-244. DOI: 10.1021/bk-2015-1211.ch008

[14] Chew SC. The southeast Asian connection in the first Eurasian world economy 200 BC AD 500. In: Hall T, editor. Comparing Globalizations. World-Systems Evolution and Global Futures. Cham, Switzerland: Springer; 2018. pp. 91-117. DOI: 10.1007/978-3-319-68219-8_5

[15] Creasman PP, Yamamoto K. The African incense trade and its impacts in pharaonic Egypt. African Archaeological Review. 2019;**36**(3):347-365. DOI: 10.1007/s10437-019-09348-8

[16] Byl SA. The Essence and Use of Perfume in Ancient Egypt. [Thesis]. Pretoria, Gauteng: University of South Africa; 2012

[17] Jones EA. Awaken to Healing Fragrance: The Power of Essential Oil Therapy. Berkeley, California: North Atlantic Books; 2010

[18] Agnihotry S et al. Aromatherapy evolution and blending basics of essential oils. Aromatherapy: The Science of Essential Oils. 2024;**1**:1-30. DOI: 10.2174/9789815136203124010005

[19] Damian P, Damian K. Aromatherapy: Scent and psyche: Using essential oils for physical and emotional well-being. In: Inner Traditions. Rochester, Vermont: Bear and Co; 1995

[20] Hedaoo SA, Chandurkar PA. A review on aromatherapy. World Journal of Pharmaceutical Research. 2019;**8**(7):635-651

[21] McHugh J. Sandalwood and Carrion: Smell in Indian Religion and Culture. Cambridge, England: Oxford University Press; 2012. DOI: 10.1093/acprof:oso/9780199916306.003.0008

[22] Fagan GG. Bathing in Public in the Roman World. East Lansing, Michigan: University of Michigan Press; 2002. DOI: 10.3998/mpub.14923

[23] Diniz do Nascimento L et al. Bioactive natural compounds and antioxidant activity of essential oils from spice plants: New findings and potential applications. Biomolecules. 2020;**10**(7):988. DOI: 10.3390/biom10070988

[24] Jung D. Bilqīs (including history up to the 12th century). In: An Ethnography of Fragrance. Leiden: Brill; 2011. pp. 29-58. DOI: 10.1163/9789004491243_006

[25] King AH. The Musk Trade and the Near East in the Early Medieval Period. Bloomington, Indiana: Indiana University; 2007

[26] Abu-Chacra F. Trade and trade routes of the Quraysh. In: Asian Trade Routes. Oxfordshire, England: Routledge; 2013. p. 38-42. DOI: 10.4324/9780203060971-11

[27] Zohar A, Lev E. Trends in the use of perfumes and incense in the near east after the Muslim conquests. Journal of the Royal Asiatic Society. 2013;**23**(1):11-30. DOI: 10.1017/s1356186312000673

[28] Manzoor F. Concept of cosmetology and its historical background in Unani perspective. Journal of Drug Delivery and Therapeutics. 2024;**14**(4):104-107. DOI: 10.22270/jddt.v14i4.6498

[29] Başer KH. Rose mentioned in the works of scientists of the medieval east and implications in modern science. Natural Product Communications. 2017;**12**(8):1934578X1701200843. DOI: 10.1177/1934578x1701200843

[30] Kaadan AN, Khatib C. Albucasis, the notable cosmetologist... worldwide. Journal of the International Society for The History Islamic Medicine. 2016;**14-15**(27-28-29-30):84-99

[31] Vora LK et al. Essential oils for clinical aromatherapy: A comprehensive review. Journal of Ethnopharmacology. 2024;**330**:118180. DOI: 10.1016/j.jep.2024.118180

[32] Balkrishna A et al. Study of essential oil bearing plants, their composition and Ayurvedic herbalism. Journal of Essential Oil and Plant Composition Health. 2024;**5**(6):23. DOI: 10.58985/jeopc.2024.v02i01.32

[33] Yang J. Introduction to Chinese Materia Medica. Vol. 3. Singapore: World Scientific; 2013

[34] AlQurashi RZA. Abdul Samad Al-Qurashi (ASQ)–an admirable growth trajectory–Middle East to a multinational presence. In: Corporate Success Stories in the UAE: The Key Drivers behind

their Growth. Leeds, England: Emerald Publishing Limited; 2021. pp. 19-32. DOI: 10.1108/978-1-80043-578-020211002

[35] Fornari T et al. Isolation of essential oil from different plants and herbs by supercritical fluid extraction. Journal of Chromatography A. 2012;**1250**:34-48. DOI: 10.1016/j.chroma.2012.04.051

[36] Zuzarte M, Salgueiro L. Essential oils chemistry. In: Bioactive Essential Oils and Cancer. Switzerland: Springer International Publishing; 2015. pp. 19-61. DOI: 10.1007/978-3-319-19144-7_2

[37] Wang Y et al. Chemistry of citrus flavor. In: The Genus Citrus. Cambridge, Cambridgeshire, United Kingdom: Woodhead Publishing; 2020. pp. 447-470. DOI: 10.1016/b978-0-12-812163-4.00022-x

[38] Eddin LB et al. Health benefits, pharmacological effects, molecular mechanisms, and therapeutic potential of α-bisabolol. Nutrients. 2022;**14**(7):1370. DOI: 10.3390/nu14071370

[39] Margetts J. Aroma chemicals V: Natural aroma chemicals. In: Chemistry and Technology of Flavors and Fragrances. Oxford, UK: Blackwell Publishing; 2005. pp. 169-198. DOI: 10.1002/9781444305517.ch8

[40] Rowe DJ. Aroma chemicals I: C, H, O compounds. In: Chemistry and Technology of Flavors and Fragrances. Oxford, UK: Blackwell Publishing Ltd; 2005. pp. 56-84. DOI: 10.1002/9781444305517.ch4

[41] Atkinson RG. Phenylpropenes: Occurrence, distribution, and biosynthesis in fruit. Journal of Agricultural and Food Chemistry. 2016;**66**(10):2259-2272. DOI: 10.1021/acs.jafc.6b04696

[42] Figueiredo AC et al. Factors affecting secondary metabolite production in plants: Volatile components and essential oils. Flavour and Fragrance Journal. 2008;**23**(4):213-226. DOI: 10.1002/ffj.1875

[43] Rocha F, Ratola N, Homem V. Fragrances in the environment: Properties, applications, and emissions. In: Ratola N, Homem V, editors. The Handbook of Environmental Chemistry. Vol. 128. Cham: Springer; 2023. DOI: 10.1007/698_2023_983

[44] Riad N et al. Occurrence of marine ingredients in fragrance: Update on the state of knowledge. Chemistry. 2021;**3**(4):1437-1463. DOI: 10.3390/chemistry3040103

[45] Butnariu M. Plants as source of essential oils and perfumery applications. In: Bioprospecting of Plant Biodiversity for Industrial Molecules. Hoboken, NJ, United States: John Wiley & Sons Ltd; 2021. pp. 261-292. DOI: 10.1002/9781119718017.ch13

[46] Michalak M. The use of carrier oils in aromatherapy massage and their effect on skin. Archives of Physiotherapy and Global Researches. 2018;**22**(3):23-31

[47] Price S, Price L. Carrier oils. In: Aromatherapy for Health Professionals Revised Reprint E-Book. Amsterdam, The Netherlands: Elsevier Limited; 2021. p. 151

[48] Afriani L et al. Aromatherapy candles as double protection: A modern solution to a classic problem. IJESS International Journal of Education and Social Science. 2024;**5**(1):155-160

[49] Li JJ et al. Effect of food emulsifiers on aroma release. Molecules. 2016;**21**(4):511. DOI: 10.3390/molecules21040511

[50] Al-Bayati ADJ. Comparative study for the effect of fixative material type and perfume formulation parameters on the fixation time of local formulated perfume with brand perfumes. Engineering And Technology Journal. 2016;**34**:636-647. DOI: 10.30684/etj.34.3a.17

[51] Poucher WA. Odour classification and fixation. In: Perfumes, Cosmetics and Soaps: Volume II. Dordrecht: Springer Netherlands; 1993. pp. 46-67. DOI: 10.1007/978-94-011-1484-4_4

[52] Hazell S. A guide to understanding deodorant formulations. In: Cosmetic Science and Technology Series. Boca Raton, Florida: CRC Press; 1999. p. 259-282. DOI: 10.1201/b15205-11

[53] Niebler J. Incense materials. In: Springer Handbook of Odor. Berlin: Springer; 2017. pp. 13-14. DOI: 10.1007/978-3-319-26932-0_4

[54] Kinkele T. Incense and Incense Rituals. Wisconsin, United States: Lotus Press; 2023

[55] Marriott PJ, Shellie R, Cornwell C. Gas chromatographic technologies for the analysis of essential oils. Journal of Chromatography A. 2001;**936**(1-2):1-22. DOI: 10.1016/s0021-9673(01)01314-0

[56] Sadgrove NJ, Padilla-González GF, Phumthum M. Fundamental chemistry of essential oils and volatile organic compounds, methods of analysis and authentication. Plants. 2022;**11**(6):789. DOI: 10.3390/plants11060789

[57] Baser KH. Analysis and quality assessment of essential oils. In: A Manual on the Essential Oil Industry. Vienna, Austria: United Nations Industrial Development Organization; 1995. p. 155

[58] Benavides J, Rojas J, Lopera Y. Instrumental analysis of flavors and fragrances in food processing: Hyphenated techniques. In: Flavors and Fragrances in Food Processing: Preparation and Characterization Methods. Washington, D.C.: American Chemical Society; 2022. pp. 341-359. DOI: 10.1021/bk-2022-1433.ch008

[59] Do TK et al. Authenticity of essential oils. TrAC Trends in Analytical Chemistry. 2015;**66**:146-157. DOI: 10.1016/j.trac.2014.10.007

[60] Rossiter KJ. Structure-odor relationships. Chemical Reviews. 1996;**96**(8):3201-3240. DOI: 10.1021/cr950068a

[61] Teixeira MA et al. Perfumery radar: A predictive tool for perfume family classification. Industrial and Engineering Chemistry Research. 2010;**49**(22):11764-11777. DOI: 10.1021/ie101161v

[62] Darden J. The Development of Novel Methods for Assessing Human Olfaction Ability and the Odor Intensity of Samples. [Master's Thesis]. Tempe, Arizona, United States: Arizona State University; 2023

[63] Urdapilleta I et al. The mental context for the description of odors: A semantic space. European Review of Applied Psychology. 2006;**56**(4):261-271. DOI: 10.1016/j.erap.2005.09.013

[64] Cortez-Pereira CS, Baby AR, Velasco MVR. Fragrance technology for the dermatologist–a review and practical application. Journal of Cosmetic Dermatology. 2010;**9**(3):230-241. DOI: 10.1111/j.1473-2165.2010.00514.x

[65] Shepherd GM. Smell images and the flavour system in the human brain. Nature. 2006;**444**(7117):316-321. DOI: 10.1038/nature05405

[66] Moshayedi AJ et al. E-nose design and structures from statistical analysis to application in robotic: A comprehensive review. EAI Endorsed Transactions on AI and Robotics. 2023;**2**:1-20. DOI: 10.4108/airo.v2i1.3056

[67] Zarzo M. Multivariate analysis of olfactory profiles for 140 perfumes as a basis to derive a sensory wheel for the classification of feminine fragrances. Cosmetics. 2020;**7**(1):11. DOI: 10.3390/cosmetics7010011

[68] Sell C. Perfumery material of natural origin. In: The Chemistry of Fragrances: From Perfumer to Consumer. 2nd ed. London: Royal Society of Chemistry; 2006. pp. 24-27. DOI: 10.1039/9781847555342-fp015

[69] González-Minero FJ, Bravo-Díaz L, Moreno-Toral E. Pharmacy and fragrances: Traditional and current use of plants and their extracts. Cosmetics. 2023;**10**(6):157. DOI: 10.3390/cosmetics10060157

[70] Rodrigues AE, Nogueira I, Faria RPV. Perfume and flavor engineering: A chemical engineering perspective. Molecules. 2021;**26**(11):3095. DOI: 10.3390/molecules26113095

[71] Boelens M, Boelens R. Classification of perfumes and fragrances. Perfumer and Flavorist. 2001;**26**(6):28-39

[72] Verlet N. Commercialization of essential oils and aroma chemicals. In: A Manual on the Essential Oil Industry. Vienna, Austria: United Nations Industrial Development Organization; 1995. pp. 228-230

[73] Nikitina L, Furuoka F. Words of scents: A linguistic analysis of online perfume reviews. Linguistics Vanguard. 2024;**9**(1):205-214. DOI: 10.1515/lingvan-2022-0135

[74] Teixeira MA et al. Perfumery radar 2.0: A step toward fragrance design and classification. Industrial and Engineering Chemistry Research. 2014;**53**(21):8890-8912. DOI: 10.1021/ie403968w

[75] Ramsbotham J. Perfumes in detergents. In: Handbook of Detergents, Part A. Boca Raton, Florida: CRC Press; 1999. pp. 691-720. DOI: 10.1201/b10985-20

[76] Sharmeen JB, Mahomoodally FM, Zengin G, Maggi F. Essential oils as natural sources of fragrance compounds for cosmetics and cosmeceuticals. Molecules. 2021;**26**(5):1187. DOI: 10.3390/molecules26030666

[77] Horváth G, Ács K. Essential oils in the treatment of respiratory tract diseases highlighting their role in bacterial infections and their anti-inflammatory action: A review. Flavour and Fragrance Journal. 2015;**30**(5):331-341. DOI: 10.1002/ffj.3252

[78] Cheema HS, Singh MP. The use of medicinal plants in digestive system related disorders—A systematic review. The Journal of Ayurveda and Integrative Medicine. 2021;**7**(3):182-187. DOI: 10.31254/jahm.2021.7303

[79] Buckle J. Use of aromatherapy as a complementary treatment for chronic pain. Alternative Therapies in Health and Medicine. 1999;**5**(5):42

[80] Verma SK, Garg AK, Singh M, Panwar N, Meena M, Singh C. Evaluation of Analgesic Activity of Syzygium Aromaticum w. sr t.

[81] Grazul M, Kwiatkowski P, Hartman K, Kilanowicz A, Sienkiewicz M. How to naturally support the immune system in inflammation—Essential oils as immune

boosters. Biomedicine. 2023;**11**(9):2381. DOI: 10.3390/biomedicines11092381

[82] Ebani VV, Nardoni S, Bertelloni F, Pistelli L, Mancianti F. Antimicrobial activity of five essential oils against bacteria and fungi responsible for urinary tract infections. Molecules. 2018;**23**(7):1668. DOI: 10.3390/molecules23071668

[83] Reichling J. Antiviral and virucidal properties of essential oils and isolated compounds–a scientific approach. Planta Medica. 2022;**88**(08):587-603. DOI: 10.1055/a-1382-2898

[84] Wei YX, Xu XY, Song X. A review of antifungal natural products against the pathogenic fungi causing athletes' foot disease. Current Organic Chemistry. 2017;**21**(18):1907-1919. DOI: 10.2174/1385272821666170206163047

[85] Farahani MA, Afsargharehbagh R, Marandi F, Moradi M, Hashemi SM, Poodineh Moghadam M, et al. Effect of aromatherapy on cancer complications: A systematic review. Complementary Therapies in Medicine. 2019;**47**:102169. DOI: 10.1016/j.ctim.2019.08.003

[86] Najar B, Shortrede JE, Pistelli L, Buhagiar J. Chemical composition and in vitro cytotoxic screening of sixteen commercial essential oils on five cancer cell lines. Chemistry and Biodiversity. 2020;**17**(1):e1900478. DOI: 10.1002/cbdv.201900478

[87] Arabatzis S. Study of Mechanisms of Cell Death Induction by the Essential Oil Aloysia Citriodora and its Major Component, Citral, and Evaluation of their Potential Synergistic Effects with Oxaliplatin in Human Colon Cancer Cells. [Thesis]. 2017

[88] Pouyamanesh G, Ameli N, Metanat Y, Khorrami A, Abbasinezhad-Moud F, Qoorchi Moheb Seraj F, et al. Thymol enhances 5-fluorouracil cytotoxicity by reducing migration and increasing apoptosis and cell cycle arrest in esophageal cancer cells: An in vitro study. Indian Journal of Clinical Biochemistry. 2024;**39**(2):1-12. DOI: 10.1007/s12291-024-01219-7

[89] Karki N. Inhibitory Activity of Ginger Oil against Breast Cancer Cells. [Thesis]. Baton Rouge, Louisiana: Louisiana State University and Agricultural and Mechanical College; 2011. DOI: 10.31390/gradschool_theses.1714

[90] Khan H, Ullah H, Castilho PCM, Sureda Gomila A, D'Onofrio G, Filosa R, et al. Targeting NF-κB signaling pathway in cancer by dietary polyphenols. Critical Reviews in Food Science and Nutrition. 2020;**60**(16):2790-2800. DOI: 10.1080/10408398.2019.1661827

[91] Angelucci FL, Silva V, Dal Pizzol C, Spir LG, Praes CEO, Maibach H. Physiological effect of olfactory stimuli inhalation in humans: An overview. International Journal of Cosmetic Science. 2014;**36**(2):117-123. DOI: 10.1111/ics.12096

[92] Dias P et al. Aromatherapy in the control of stress and anxiety. Alternative and Integrative Medicine. 2017;**6**:1-5. DOI: 10.4172/2327-5162.1000248

[93] Hur MH et al. Aromatherapy for stress reduction in healthy adults: A systematic review and meta-analysis of randomized clinical trials. Maturitas. 2014;**79**(4):362-369. DOI: 10.1016/j.maturitas.2014.08.006

[94] Diego MA, Jones NA, Field T, Hernandez-Reif M, Schanberg S, Kuhn C, et al. Aromatherapy positively affects mood, EEG patterns of alertness and math computations.

International Journal of Neuroscience. 1998;**96**(3-4):217-224. DOI: 10.3109/00207459808986469

[95] Yang CP, Yang CC, Tsai IJ, Lin TH, Chiou YL, Wang HF, et al. The immediate effects of lavender-based essential oil inhalation on subsequent polysomnography in people with poor sleep quality. Journal of the Chinese Medical Association. 2023;**86**(7):665-671. DOI: 10.1097/jcma.0000000000000932

[96] Thompson S. Spiritual practice and essential oil therapy: Exploring the history and individual preferences among specific plant sources. International Journal of Aromatherapy. 2003;**13**(2-3):108-113. DOI: 10.1016/s0962-4562(03)00096-1

[97] Barnett JE, Shale AJ. The integration of complementary and alternative medicine (CAM) into the practice of psychology: A vision for the future. Professional Psychology: Research and Practice. 2012;**43**(6):576. DOI: 10.1037/a0028919

[98] Capellini S. The complete spa book for massage therapists. Milady/Cengage Learning. 2010:19-45

[99] Edris AE. Pharmaceutical and therapeutic potentials of essential oils and their individual volatile constituents: A review. Phytotherapy Research. 2007;**21**(4):308-323. DOI: 10.1002/ptr.2072

[100] Rowland E. The Healing Power of Scent: A beginner's Guide to the Power of Essential Oils. Exeter, England: David and Charles; 2024

[101] Bunse M, Daniels R, Gründemann C, Heilmann J, Kammerer DR, Keusgen M, et al. Essential oils as multicomponent mixtures and their potential for human health and well-being. Frontiers in Pharmacology. 2022;**13**:956541. DOI: 10.3389/fphar.2022.956541

[102] Ande SN, Bakal RL. Potential herbal essential oils: Are they super natural skin protectors. Innova Pharmactive. 2022;**10**:19-24

[103] Guzmán E, Lucia A. Essential oils and their individual components in cosmetic products. Cosmetics. 2021;**8**(4):114. DOI: 10.3390/cosmetics8040114

[104] Chinnappan S, Wong SY, Liow YM, Tan ZJ, Tham JL, Panneerselvam J, et al. Natural essential oils for antiaging: A review. Research Journal of Pharmacy and Technology. 2024;**17**(5):2398-2404. DOI: 10.52711/0974-360x.2024.00375

[105] Nascimento T, Gomes D, Simões R, Miguel MG. Tea tree oil: Properties and the therapeutic approach to acne—A review. Antioxidants. 2023;**12**(6):1264. DOI: 10.3390/antiox12061264

[106] Blaak J, Staib P. An updated review on efficacy and benefits of sweet almond, evening primrose and jojoba oils in skin care applications. International Journal of Cosmetic Science. 2022;**44**(1):1-9. DOI: 10.1111/ics.12758

[107] Abelan US, Oliveira AC, Cacoci ES, Martins TEA, Giacon VM, Velasco MVR, et al. Potential use of essential oils in cosmetic and dermatological hair products: A review. Journal of Cosmetic Dermatology. 2022;**21**(4):1407-1418. DOI: 10.1111/jocd.14286

[108] Lee BH, Lee JS, Kim YC. Hair growth-promoting effects of lavender oil in C57BL/6 mice. Toxicological Research. 2016;**32**:103-108. DOI: 10.5487/tr.2016.32.2.103

[109] Leite Junior AC, Bastos CCB. Essential oils for hair health: A critical

mini-review of the current evidence and future directions. Brazilian Journal of Aromatherapy and Essential Oil. 2024;**1**(1):1-9. DOI: 10.62435/2965-7253.bjhae.2024.bjhae3

[110] Kumari KM, Yadav N, Luqman S. Promising essential oils/plant extracts in the prevention and treatment of dandruff pathogenesis. Current Topics in Medicinal Chemistry. 2022;**22**(13):1104-1133. DOI: 10.2174/156802662266622053 1120226

[111] Patel SD. A review of herbal cosmetics used for skin care and hair care. Life Sciences Leaflets. 2024;**171**:1-23

[112] Tschiggerl C, Bucar F. The volatile fraction of herbal teas. Phytochemistry Reviews. 2012;**11**:245-254. DOI: 10.1007/s11101-012-9244-6

[113] Onaolapo AY, Onaolapo OJ. Herbal beverages and brain function in health and disease. In: Functional and Medicinal Beverages. Academic Press; 2019. pp. 313-349. DOI: 10.1016/b978-0-12-816397-9.00009-1

[114] Romics I, Siller G, Kohnen R, Mavrogenis S, Varga J, Holman E. A special terpene combination (Rowatinex®) improves stone clearance after extracorporeal shockwave lithotripsy in urolithiasis patients: Results of a placebo-controlled randomised controlled trial. Urologia Internationalis. 2011;**86**(1):102-109. DOI: 10.1159/000320999

[115] Matera R, Lucchi E, Valgimigli L. Plant essential oils as healthy functional ingredients of nutraceuticals and diet supplements: A review. Molecules. 2023;**28**(2):901. DOI: 10.3390/molecules28020901

[116] Tongnuanchan P, Benjakul S. Essential oils: Extraction, bioactivities, and their uses for food preservation. Journal of Food Science. 2014;**79**(7):R1231-R1249. DOI: 10.1111/1750-3841.12492

[117] Martin I. Aromatherapy for massage practitioners. Lippincott Williams and Wilkins. 2007:29-31

[118] Aswandi A, Kholibrina CR, Kuspradini H. Essential oils for cosmetics application. In: Biomass-Based Cosmetics: Research Trends and Future Outlook. Singapore: Springer Nature Singapore; 2024. pp. 151-173. DOI: 10.1007/978-981-97-1908-2_7

[119] White J, Downers K. Aromatherapy for Scentual Awareness. Bloomington, Indiana, United States: Balboa Press; 2011

[120] Manoharan P, Kaliaperumal K. Salt and skin. International Journal of Dermatology. 2022;**61**(3):291-298. DOI: 10.1111/ijd.15588

[121] Keller E. Aromatherapy Handbook for Beauty, Hair, and Skin Care. Rochester, Vermont: Inner Traditions/Bear and Co; 1999

[122] Tavares CS, Gameiro JA, Roseiro LB, Figueiredo AC. Hydrolates: A review on their volatiles composition, biological properties and potential uses. Phytochemistry Reviews. 2022;**21**(5):1661-1737. DOI: 10.1007/s11101-022-09803-6

[123] Du B, Schwartz-Narbonne H, Tandoc M, Heffernan EM, Mack ML, Siegel JA. The impact of emissions from an essential oil diffuser on cognitive performance. Indoor Air. 2022;**32**(1):e12919. DOI: 10.1111/ina.12919

[124] Gurkok S, Sezen S. Uses of essential oils in different sectors. In: Essential Oils:

Extraction Methods and Applications. Beverly Hills, California: Scrivener Publishing LLC; 2023. pp. 207-228. DOI: 10.1002/9781119829614.ch10

[125] West A, Annett-Hitchcock K. The development of an herb-infused bag that regenerates aromatherapy textiles. International Journal of Designed Objects. 2016;**10**(2):17-30. DOI: 10.18848/2325-1379/cgp/v10i02/17-30

[126] Varney E, Buckle J. Effect of inhaled essential oils on mental exhaustion and moderate burnout: A small pilot study. The Journal of Alternative and Complementary Medicine. 2013;**19**(1):69-71. DOI: 10.1089/acm.2012.0089

[127] Panda S, Sahoo S, Tripathy K, Singh YD, Sarma MK, Babu PJ, et al. Essential oils and their pharmacotherapeutics applications in human diseases. Advances in Traditional Medicine. 2020;**22**(2022):1-15. DOI: 10.1007/s13596-020-00477-z

[128] Halligudi N, Al OM. The science and art of aromatherapy: A brief review. Journal of Biomedical and Pharmaceutical Research. 2013;**2**(2):6-14

[129] Yadav VK, Choudhary N, Khan SH, Khayal A, Ravi RK, Kumar P, et al. Incense and incense sticks: Types, components, origin and their religious beliefs and importance among different religions. Journal of Bio Innovation. 2020;**9**:1420-1439. DOI: 10.46344/jbino.2020.v09i06.28

[130] Burger P, Plainfossé H, Brochet X, Chemat F, Fernandez X. Extraction of natural fragrance ingredients: History overview and future trends. Chemistry and Biodiversity. 2019;**16**(10):e1900424. DOI: 10.1002/cbdv.201900424

[131] Mensing J. Scent therapy: Scents for more joie de vivre: Working with primal perfumes in scent-assisted therapy—A look into the future at what else might be possible for increasing well-being. In: Beautiful SCENT: The Magical Effect of Perfume on Well-Being. Berlin, Heidelberg: Springer Berlin Heidelberg; 2023. pp. 223-253. DOI: 10.1007/978-3-662-67259-4_10

[132] Narula APS. The search for new fragrance ingredients for functional perfumery perspectives in flavor and fragrance research. In: Chemistry & Biodiversity. Zürich: Verlag Helvetica Chimica Acta; 2004. pp. 1992-1994. DOI: 10.1002/9783906390475.ch14

[133] Shanthi V, Diwan S. Application of essential oils in industries and daily usage. In: Essential Oils: Sources, Production and Applications. Berlin, Boston: De Gruyter; 2023. pp. 155-157. DOI: 10.1515/9783110791600-008

[134] Pageau A. Tinctures for use in aromatherapy. Aromatherapy Journal. 2020;**2020**(4):73-78

[135] Vostinaru O, Heghes SC, Filip L. Safety profile of essential oils. In: Essential Oils-Bioactive Compounds, New Perspectives and Applications. London, UK: IntechOpen; 2020. pp. 1-13. DOI: 10.5772/intechopen.91363

[136] De Groot AC, Frosch PJ. Adverse reactions to fragrances: A clinical review. Contact Dermatitis. 1997;**36**(2):57-86. DOI: 10.1111/j.1600-0536.1997.tb00418.x

[137] Schaller M, Korting HC. Allergie airborne contact dermatitis from essential oils used in aromatherapy. Clinical and Experimental Dermatology. 1995;**20**(2):143-145. DOI: 10.1111/j.1365-2230.1995.tb02719.x

[138] Shukla A, Kushwaha A, Sanju S, Spring P, Kumar A, Misra P, et al. Essential oils toxicity and conflicts.

In: Aromatherapy: The Science of Essential Oils. Netherlands: Bentham Science Publishers; 2024. p. 124. DOI: 10.2174/9789815136203124010009

[139] Manion CR, Widder RM. Essentials of essential oils. American Journal of Health-System Pharmacy. 2017;**74**(9):e153-e162. DOI: 10.2146/ajhp151043

[140] Williamson EM. Drug interactions between herbal and prescription medicines. Drug Safety. 2003;**26**:1075-1092. DOI: 10.2165/00002018-200326150-00002

[141] Abebe W. Review of herbal medications with the potential to cause bleeding: Dental implications, and risk prediction and prevention avenues. EPMA Journal. 2019;**10**:51-64. DOI: 10.1007/s13167-018-0158-2

[142] Poppenga RH. Herbal medicine: Potential for intoxication and interactions with conventional drugs. Clinical Techniques in Small Animal Practice. 2002;**17**(1):6-18. DOI: 10.1053/svms.2002.27785

[143] Cadby PA, Troy WR, Vey MGH. Consumer exposure to fragrance ingredients: Providing estimates for safety evaluation. Regulatory Toxicology and Pharmacology. 2002;**36**(3):246-252. DOI: 10.1006/rtph.2002.1581

[144] Boyer IJ, Bergfeld WF, Heldreth B, Fiume MM, Gill LJ. The cosmetic ingredient review program—Expert safety assessments of cosmetic ingredients in an open forum. International Journal of Toxicology. 2017;**36**(5_suppl2):5S-13S. DOI: 10.1177/1091581817717646

[145] Michailidou F. The scent of change: Sustainable fragrances through industrial biotechnology. Chembiochem. 2023;**24**(19):e202300309. DOI: 10.1002/cbic.202300309

[146] Waseem R, Low KH. Advanced analytical techniques for the extraction and characterization of plant-derived essential oils by gas chromatography with mass spectrometry. Journal of Separation Science. 2015;**38**(3):483-501. DOI: 10.1002/jssc.201400724

[147] Smelcerovic A, Djordjevic A, Lazarevic J, Stojanovic G. Recent advances in analysis of essential oils. Current Analytical Chemistry. 2013;**9**(1):61-70. DOI: 10.2174/157341113804486464

[148] Saifullah M, Shishir MRI, Ferdowsi R, Rahman MRT, Vuong QV. Micro and nano encapsulation, retention and controlled release of flavor and aroma compounds: A critical review. Trends in Food Science and Technology. 2019;**86**:230-251. DOI: 10.1016/j.tifs.2019.02.030

[149] Żukowska G, Durczyńska Z. Properties and applications of essential oils: A review. Journal of. Ecological Engineering. 2024;**25**(2):333-340. DOI: 10.12911/22998993/177404

[150] Wang M, Wang W, Zhang X, Dai G, Tang K. Formulation analysis of functional fragrance via polar-gradient extraction method and chemometrics pattern recognition. Talanta. 2024;**275**:126121. DOI: 10.1016/j.talanta.2024.126121

[151] Nalla S, Golla U, Palatheeya S, Aouta EK. Aromatherapy: An integrative therapy of essential oils. In: Pharmacological Aspects of Essential Oils. Boca Raton, FL, USA: CRC Press; 2024. pp. 120-125. DOI: 10.1201/9781003389774-8

[152] Collu M. New Methodologies for Environmentally Friendly Microcapsule

Design. [Thesis]. Barcelona, Spain: Universitat Rovira i Virgili; 2024

[153] Altay Ö, Köprüalan Ö, İlter I, Koç M, Kaymak Ertekin F, Jafari SM. Spray drying encapsulation of essential oils; process efficiency, formulation strategies, and applications. Critical Reviews in Food Science and Nutrition. 2024;**64**(4):1139-1157. DOI: 10.1080/10408398.2022.2113364

[154] Zhang L, Lin J, Zhang C, Hu S, Dong Y, Fan G, et al. Recent advances in the nanotechnology-based applications of essential oils. Current Nanoscience. 2024;**20**(5):630-643. DOI: 10.2174/15734 13719666230718122527

[155] Yap XF, Saw SH, Lim V, Tan CX. Plant essential oil nanoemulgel as a cosmeceutical ingredient: A review. Cosmetics. 2024;**11**(4):116. DOI: 10.3390/cosmetics11040116

[156] Andriansyah M, Zaini H. Making aroma fragrance gel using carrageenan and pectin with lemon oil (Citrus Limon) fragrance. Chelo Journal of Technological Development of Engineering (CEJOTER). 2024;**1**(2):53-62

[157] Katare P, Polaka S, Nalla LV, Makwana V, Tekade RK. Insect repellents as an environmental chemical toxicant to human health. In: Public Health and Toxicology Issues Drug Research. Volume 2. Cambridge, Massachusetts: Academic Press; 2024. pp. 523-554. DOI: 10.1016/b978-0-443-15842-1.00003-x

[158] Xin H, Virk AS, Virk SS, Akin-Ige F, Amin S. Applications of artificial intelligence and machine learning on critical materials used in cosmetics and personal care formulation design. Current Opinion in Colloid and Interface Science. 2024;**73**:101847. DOI: 10.1016/j.cocis.2024.101847

[159] Lee J, Kwon K. Future challenges of direct-to-consumer genetic testing for sustainable safety in the Republic of Korea's skin care market: A systematic review. mHealth. 2024;**1**:1-15. DOI: 10.21037/mhealth-23-61

[160] Sasounian R, Martinez RM, Lopes AM, Giarolla J, Rosado C, Magalhães WV, et al. Innovative approaches to an eco-friendly cosmetic industry: A review of sustainable ingredients. Clean Technologies. 2024;**6**(1):176-198. DOI: 10.3390/cleantechnol6010011

[161] Rantala J, Salminen K, Isokoski P, Nieminen V, Karjalainen M, Väliaho J, et al. Recall of odorous objects in virtual reality. Multimodal Technologies and Interaction. 2024;**8**(6):42. DOI: 10.3390/mti8060042

[162] Cicconi S. Augmented Total Theatre: Shaping the Future of Immersive Augmented Reality Representations. i-com. 2024. DOI: 10.1515/icom-2024-0011

[163] Tewell J, Ranasinghe N. A review of olfactory display designs for virtual reality environments. ACM Computing Surveys. 2024;**56**(11):1-35. DOI: 10.1145/3665243

Chapter 6

New Prospects of Alternative Medicine from Plant Sources in Management of Alzheimer's Disease

Daisy Jepkosgei Kipkemoi

Abstract

Although the cure for Alzheimer's disease (AD) remains elusive, the scientific community has remained vigilant in search of remedies for AD management. The statistics in the fight against AD paint a pale picture; the number of people suffering from Alzheimer's disease remains high. About 40 million people worldwide, mainly the elderly, are experiencing AD and the number is expected to rise in the next decade. Meanwhile, FDA-certified drugs for AD management only relieve symptoms of the disease and provide a limited benefit to the cognitive functioning of the patient. The increasing economic and social burden as well as drawbacks of the current AD management measures highlights the need for urgent attention in search of alternative avenues to combat AD. A major area of focus in this endeavour is herbal therapy. Universally, humanity appreciably recognizes the role herbal medicines have played in catering to human health. Presently, 80% of the global populace relies on plant-based remedies for primary healthcare. Numerous herbal preparations have been reported to exhibit anti-AD efficacy in various research models. This chapter provides an account of AD pathophysiology and various herbal preparations with efficacy against AD in various study models: clinical trials, *in vivo*, *in vitro* and *in silico*.

Keywords: Alzheimer's disease, clinical trials, *in vivo*, *in vitro*, *in silico*, herbal therapy

1. Introduction

Alzheimer's disease (AD) also known as pre-senile dementia, is a mental disorder characterized by severe memory loss, behavior, personality and cognitive dysfunction [1, 2]. The condition begins as mild with no or minimal amnestic symptoms then progresses gradually through moderate to severity stages when symptoms are well established. The rise of severe symptoms may occur approximately 20 years or more after the onset of the disease [3]. Clinically AD patients suffer severe memory impairment, language complications, discoordination, cognitive and reasoning deficits. Psychiatric manifestations of AD include delusions, hallucinations, anxiety, apathy, irritation and depression [4]. As the cognitive faculties continue to deteriorate, the patient loses the ability to carry out daily tasks essential to live an effective and fulfilling life. Sadly, eventually, mortality occurs partly due to compounded effects among them, infections, dysphagia and starvation [5]. The precise mechanism of AD remains unclear due to multiple physiological hallmarks. Amyloid β plaques and over-phosphorylated tau protein are the two toxins that are known to cause neuronal cell death in AD pathology. Besides, decrease in acetylcholine, increased oxidative stress, bio-metal dysregulation and neuroinflammation can aggravate AD pathogenesis [1, 6].

The patient zero for AD was Auguste Deter, a 51-year-old lady diagnosed by Dr. Alois Alzheimer in 1901 [2]. Since then, the statistics for AD have continued to rise. AD is recognized as the most prevalent and detrimental type of neurological illness [7]. It accounts for about 80% of all dementia cases globally. Of the 50 million global cases of dementia, 45–47 million are caused by AD, and this statistic is anticipated to rise threefold by 2050 [1, 7]. Further, the treatment of AD together with other types of dementia is among the most expensive and economically burdening diseases of the twenty-first Century [6]. The annual cost of healthcare for AD is at US dollars 1.3 trillion and is anticipated to rise to USD 2.8 trillion before the year 2030 [8]. Consequently, there is an urgent necessity to develop initiatives to avert the progression of AD.

There are various mainstay therapies for Alzheimer's disease including donepezil, rivastigmine, memantine and galantamine [9]. Though widely used, these orthodox therapies are not without recognized shortcomings. The drugs are known to only alleviate symptoms instead of curing the disease, hence, there is no known curative agent for Alzheimer's to date. Besides, these remedies are marred with poor efficacy and side effects [10]. Further, they are costly resulting in a significant economic burden. The limitations of modern therapy in combating AD have motivated the focus of drug research to traditional herbal medicine. In search of new therapies for Alzheimer's disease, plant-derived alternatives have been a promising advent [11]. Indeed, plants have been a friend of mankind as a source of diet and relief since the dawn of human civilization. One of the oldest records of indigenous knowledge on herbal medicine, the Shen Nongs Medical Herbal Book, goes back as far as 3000 BC [12]. Up-to-date, well-established traditional medicine systems including Ayurveda, Kampo, Hanbang and Chinese herbal medicine continue to play a major role in modern medicine [11, 13]. Some products identified through these systems are already in clinical use while others serve as lead molecules for drug development [14].

World Health Organization estimates that 70–80% of the global populace utilizes folklore medicine as a source of health care [15]. In particular, 4 billion individuals worldwide use herbal medicines. The publicity that herbal medicine has accrued could be accredited to several beneficial outcomes [16]. Herbal extracts, due to the synergy of all their constituents, are considered better in terms of efficacy compared to synthetically derived monotherapies. Plant extracts act as multidrug with multi-targets in a biological system [17]. As a result, the paradigm is shifting toward the use of medicinal plants for the treatment of many human illnesses as modern medicine is focusing on multidrug remedies [18]. Cost is another considerable attribute that has shifted the popularity gradient toward herbal therapeutics. While conventional therapies are expensive and mostly imported to many emerging economies, herbal remedies are locally available, easily accessible and pocket-friendly [19]. The populace around the globe is impressed with the natural source of herbal remedies which is compounds by their safety and limited side effects [19]. Though, effective, conventional therapy struggles with unwanted side effects [16].

Plants have been observed to act as nootropic agents with the capability to enhance cognitive functionalities [20]. They have diverse mechanisms of action involving modulation of hormones, neurotransmitters and enzymes that control brain health and activity [21]. Some herbs enhance the release of phosphatidylinositol, acetylcholine, glutamine and dopamine essential for brain activity [22]. Also, herbal remedies are seen to increase the blood flow to the brain supplying it with essential nutrients, energy resources and adequate oxygen, consequently refining its cognitive output [23]. Medicinal plant formulations with nootropic properties are being considered for the management of cognitive deficits and neurodegenerative disorders. The application of herbal remedies in the management of neuronal anomalies is common practice in traditional medicine [24, 25]. Plant-derived medicinal products are intensively being investigated for their ability to improve neuronal functions and alleviate neurological disorders. Particularly, many medicinal plants exhibiting outstanding therapeutic potency against AD have been reported [26]. This chapter expounds on the emerging trends in the efficacies of plant-derived agents in the management of Alzheimer's disease with a central focus on clinical trials.

2. Methodology

Literature was retrieved from online databases containing academic literature: Google Scholar, PubMed, Web of Science, ProQuest, Clinical Trials.org, Science Direct and various peer-reviewed journals. Literature search combined various keywords and search strategies; "Alzheimer* Disease" AND ("Plant Extract*" OR "Medicinal Plants" OR "herbal extracts" OR "Herbal drugs"). ((("Alzheimer Disease" [Mesh]) AND ("Alzheimer Disease/drug therapy"[Mesh] OR "Alzheimer Disease/diet therapy" [Mesh] OR "Alzheimer Disease/pathology" [Mesh] "prevention and control" [Mesh] OR "Alzheimer Disease/therapy"[Mesh])) AND "Plants, Medicinal"[Mesh]) AND ("Herbal Medicine"[Mesh] OR "Drugs, Chinese Herbal"[Mesh] AND "Phytotherapy"[Mesh] OR "Plant Extracts"[Mesh]). "Alzheimer* Disease" AND "Plant Extracts" OR "Medicinal Plants" OR "herbal extracts" OR "Herbal drugs". "Research article" AND ("medicinal plants" OR "herbal") AND "Alzheimer's disease". "Alzheimer Disease" AND "Research article" AND "Plants, Medicinal" AND "Plant Extracts". "Alzheimer* Disease" AND ("Plant Extract*" OR "Medicinal Plants" OR "herbal extracts" OR "Herbal drugs"). "Clinical trial" AND "Alzheimer* Disease" AND ("Plant Extract*" OR "Medicinal Plants" OR "herbal extracts" OR "Herbal drugs"). The retrieved articles were reviewed and research articles written in English language, all-text, clinical trials, *in silico, in vitro* and *in vivo* were eligible to be included. *In vivo, in silico* and *in vitro* published before 2020 and clinical trials published before 2015 were excluded from the study.

3. Molecular basis of AD

Molecularly, AD's pathogenies occur via multifaceted pathways. Numerous hypotheses have been sought to explain the onset and progression of AD. Some of the notable hypothesis include:

3.1 Amyloid beta (β) hypothesis

Production, misfolding and build-up of amyloid beta deposits (AβP) in the brain are considered the most consequential causative hallmarks of AD [27]. The AβPs are produced from aberrant processing of amyloid precursor protein (APP), a transmembrane glycoprotein largely secreted by neurons and to lesser amounts by astrocytes [1]. APP is broken down by secretase protease; α-secretase, β-secretase and γ-secretase. Under healthy homeostasis, APP is digested by α and γ-secretases to form harmless peptides where a steady state is maintained between synthesis and excretion of the fragments from the brain tissues [6]. On the other hand, in a pathological state, APP is sliced by β and γ-secretases to generate the AβPs ranging from 37 to 43 amino acid residues [6]. These fragments, particularly Aβ42, misfold and gradually aggregate to form Aβ deposits containing harmful protofibrils, oligomers, fibrils and senile plaques within the extracellular neuronal spaces [28].

Aβ deposits are destructive to neuronal cells in numerous ways. They obstruct the signaling link in the synaptic junction resulting in synaptic dysregulation and apoptosis of neural cells [6]. Ultimately, this affects signal relay through the central nervous system with ultimate damage to the neurons and decline of brain cognitive capabilities. As such, Aβ oligomers have been demonstrated to bind to glutamate receptors through which they distort synaptic plasticity and memory acquisition [29, 30]. Besides, Aβ aggregates are thought to induce other pathological states like tau over-phosphorylation, metal dysregulation, oxidative assault, mitochondrial injury, inflammation and angiopathy, all of which accelerate neuronal damage and death [6, 31].

3.2 Tau hyper-phosphorylation hypothesis

Tau protein is a component of neurons' cytoskeleton where it is involved in the assembly and stabilizing of microtubules [32]. Microtubules serve as roads for cellular transport. The protein is mainly found in the microtubules localized to the axons and the cell body. Tau anomaly is consequential to microtubule instability in the neurons. Activated kinases over-phosphorylates tau (pTau) which leads to its release from the microtubules eventually weakening them [32, 33]. Subsequently, the detached pTau associates to form intracellular clumps known as neurofibrillary tangles (NFTs) [34].

The NFTs establish the pathological state of tauopathy in AD. NFTs mediate synaptic and neuronal dysfunction which ultimately results in cognition impairment observed in AD [31]. NFT increases oxidative stress in the brain cells which halts their functionality [35]. Besides, the collapse of the cellular transport system affects metabolism and energy production in the neural cells which potentiates their death [1]. More so, microtubule instability can lead to signaling dysregulation and apoptosis of neurons. Further, the level of NFTs directly correlated with the severity of AD [1].

It is no doubt that Tau and AβP play a consequence role in AD pathology. But, is either of the two hypotheses, the tau or AβP hypothesis alone, sufficient to account for the etiology and prognosis of AD? Evidence suggests that they are interlinked, together playing a pivotal but detrimental role in the pathogenesis of AD. Of dilemma is, which of these two hypotheses initiates the AD pathology? There are lines of evidence that support the proposition that AβP induces Tauopathy in AD and vice versa [27, 36]. Recently, there has been a growing body of evidence favoring the former, that deposition of AβP in the extracellular neuronal space triggers tau pathology [37, 38]. That notwithstanding, tau deposits also occur fairly early during the onset of AD which makes them potential diagnostic and therapeutic targets in the management of AD [6, 36].

3.3 Cholinergic system hypothesis

The cholinergic system is vital for synaptic signaling and plasticity, universally; neurotransmission. It comprises the cholinergic receptors (ChR), neurotransmitter; acetylcholine (ACh), choline acetyltransferase and acetylcholinesterase (AChE) [39]. The cholinergic system utilizes acetylcholine via the cholinergic receptors to regulate neurotransmission [40]. ACh is produced from choline and acetyl coenzyme A via a reaction catalyzed by choline acetyltransferase [41]. Under normal physiology, ACh binds to ChR receptors in the synaptic gap to propagate a neuronal signal. Thereafter, AChE at the synaptic junction neutralizes the signal transmission by degrading ACh to acetic acid and choline [42].

This hypothesis describes dysregulation of the cholinergic system at the synaptic cleft of neuronal cells in the brain which results in loss of learning and memory as well as cognitive deficits [43]. Under normal conditions, the homeostasis of ACh is carefully coordinated to ensure a steady state between its synthesis and breakdown [44]. However, in AD, the equilibrium is destabilized resulting in a significant reduction of ACh below the levels required for synaptic functioning and cognitive vitality. Inhibition of ACh hydrolysis has been shown to reinstate the cholinergic system and revert the symptoms of cognitive impairment in AD patients. The cholinergic system is a therapeutic target for the drugs used in clinical practice for the management of AD [45].

3.4 Oxidative stress

Oxidative stress involves excessive generation of free radicals in the body which cause tissue and cellular damage [46]. The radicals are categorized into reactive nitrogen and oxygen species. Physiologically, the radicals are produced to help the body fight against infectious pathogens like bacteria and viruses. Pathological states kick in when their levels overwhelm the body's antioxidant mechanism which neutralizes them [46, 47]. In the unbalanced state, oxidative radicals interact with cellular biomacromolecules; lipids, proteins and DNA, producing harmful by-products. These toxicants alter the normal cellular physiological which eventually damages cells and results in their death [47].

Oxidative stress is a common phenomenon in AD state. Various factors have been associated with oxidative stress in AD. Aβ plaques and NFT aggregates are known to initiate and fuel oxidative damage of neurons in AD [48]. Aβ forms complexes with redox reactive metals; Cu and Fe, which induce redox cycling continuously generating a build-up of oxidative radicals. Further, mitochondrial dysfunction observed in AD initiates a chain of pathways that lead to the production of elevated levels of oxidative radicals [49].

The brain is the furthermost susceptible organ to oxidative stress in the body because neurons have a higher rate of oxygen expenditure [50]. Products of oxidative reactions lead to damage of protein, lipid and DNA in the brain which severely affects normal physiology and death of neuronal cells [50, 51]. For instance, 2-propenal produced from lipid peroxidation attacks neurons resulting in the blocking of ion-motive

ATPases, glial cell sodium ion-dependent glutamate, and disrupting signaling pathways, collectively killing neuronal cells [52]. Antioxidants present in numerous herbal plants and food substances have been revealed to provide symptomatic relief to AD patients [53].

4. Plant derived candidates for AD

4.1 Preclinical plant derived candidates for AD management

There has been significant investment, by the scientific community, in the study of the efficacy and safety of plant-derived materials to combat Alzheimer's disease worldwide. To date, there are numerous accounts of *in silico, in vitro* and *in vivo* efficacies of medicinal plants in AD research models. Among them, flavonoids- and dihydroxycinnamic acids-rich ethanolic fraction of *Origanum vulgare* ssp. *vulgare* exhibited anti-AChE activity and substantial antioxidant capacity, revealing the potential for the development of anti-Alzheimer's disease agents [54]. *Scutellaria baicalensis's* potency against Alzheimer's disease was demonstrated via *in silico* and *in vitro* studies which revealed that the plant components could inhibit STAT3 production by reducing the expression of PIK3R1/SRC network in Neuro 2A cells [55]. Combinations of *Evodia rutaecarpa* and *Schisandra chinensis* have been shown to enhance memory and learning in AD rat model via increased production P-TrkB, CREB and BDNF while reducing Tau protein and GSK-3β production and Aβ1-42 [56]. Blueberry extracts with high anthocyanin content enhances autophagy-lysosomal avenue and reduces neuronal harm in *in vitro* and *in vivo* AD models [57].

Cannabis sativa L. flower and bud extracts demonstrated promising anti-AD potential by inhibiting β-secretase and cholinesterase enzymes *in vitro* [58]. *Woodfordia fruticosa* and *Bergenia ciliata* extracts have been reported to enhance memory in Passive Avoidance and Morris Water Maze tests using Swiss albino mice. Besides, these extracts have been shown to block the activities of acetylcholinesterase (AChE) and butyrylcholinesterase (BChE) in vitro revealing potential as anti-AD agents [59]. Alkaloids, carbazole-type, isolated from *Murraya koenigii* demonstrated the ability to enhance neuron growth *in vitro.* The compound was used to synthesize derivatives which improved learning and memory in AD model mice [60]. *In vitro* studies revealed that polyphenolics-rich extract of *Loranthus globosus* possess significant anti-oxidant potency and inhibitory efficacy against cholinesterase, thereby emerging as a candidate for anti-AD drugs [30]. **Table 1** provides a summary of additional candidate medicinal plants with proven anti-AD efficacy;

4.2 Plant derived candidates for AD management with clinical evidence

As research on anti-AD medicinal plants is progressing in lab-based studies, some of the findings have translated into clinical research. Indeed, several plant-derived materials have demonstrated efficacy against different levels of AD in numerous clinical studies. Among others, in a 96-week clinical study, *Melissa officinalis* preparation enriched with rosmarinic acid, a natural polyphenol, was found to reduce cognitive decline among older adults with mild AD dementia [106]. Fenugreek seed extract feeding for 4 months has been indicated to improve quality of life, memory and inhibition of oxidative stress among patients with mild to moderate AD [107]. Sesame oil cake extract has been revealed to reduce plasma amyloid-β40 and amyloid-β42

No.	Name and nature of the plant extract	Activity	Model	References
1.	Essential oil components of *Citrus aurantium* leaf	Inhibition of BChE and AChE activities	*In vitro*	[61]
2.	Ethanolic and Ethyl acetate extracts *Ugni molinae* leaf	Blocking of β-amyloid Aggregation	*In vitro*	[62]
3.	*Oxalis corniculata* Linn methanolic extract	Restoring antioxidant rotection by increasing HO-1/Nrf2 hub, inhibiting neuroinflammation through the TLR4/NLRP3, halting apoptosis and reducing Aβ production, pTau, ApoE4, LRP1 and BACE1 levels. Enhancing autophagy & regulating GSK3β route.	*In vivo*	[63]
4.	Alkaloids of *Uncaria rhynchophylla*	Inhibition of Aβ and tau pathology	*In silico*	[64]
5.	Polyphenolic-rich Pine Bark extract	Reduction of Amyloid-β and Tau Misfolding	*In vitro* and *In vivo*	[65]
6.	Mulberry fruit extract	Enhances removal of amyloid-β and blocks neuroinflammation	*In vivo*	[66]
7.	Alkaloid-containing extract of *Vernonia amygdalina*	Antioxidant and anti-AChE activities	*In vitro* and *in vivo*	[67]
8.	Water and ethanolic extracts of *Euterpe oleraceae* (Acai berry)	Antioxidant and anti-cholinesterase potency	*In vitro*	[68]
9.	Crude alcoholic extract of *Pandanus amaryllifolius*	Inhibition of Aβ aggregation	*In vitro*	[69]
10.	Green coffee bean extract	Improvement of antioxidant and cortical cholinergic activity as well inhibition of amyloid plaque production	*In vivo*	[70]
11.	Phytochemicals of *Beta vulgaris* extract	Anti-AChE activities	*In silico* and *in vitro*	[71]
12.	*Allium roseum* L. extract	Inhibition of Aß42 aggregation and toxicity	*In vitro*	[72]
13.	*Ishige okamurae* extracts	Reduction of $A\beta_{25\text{-}35}$-induced cellular apoptosis and neuroinflammation via modulation of the ERK, p38 MAPK, and JNK cues	*In vitro* and *in vivo*	[73]
14.	*Andrographis paniculata* phytochemicals	Inhibition of neuroinflammation and anti-cholinesterase potency	*In silico* and *in vitro*	[74]
15.	Organic extracts of *Nelumbo nucifera*	Antioxidant, anti-BACE-1 anti-AChE and anti-BChE, capabilities	*In vitro*	[75]
16.	Aqueous extract of *Cassiae semen* and *Forsythiae fructus*	Inhibition of Aβ aggregation and hippocampal pTau	*In vivo*	[76]
17.	*Citrus sinensis* pressurized liquid extract	Anti-Aβ-peptide toxicity	*In vivo*	[77]

No.	Name and nature of the plant extract	Activity	Model	References
18.	*Ficus benghalensis* aerial root extract	Antioxidant and anti-acetylcholinesterase potency	*In vitro*	[78]
19.	Extract of *Cynomorium songaricum*	Correction of mitochondrial structural impairments and dysfunction	*In vitro*	[79]
20.	Extract of *Syzygium aromaticum* (Clove)	Antioxidant activity in human neuroblastoma	*In vitro*	[80]
21.	Root extract of *Platycodon grandiflorum*	Inhibition of Aβ deposition, oxidative stress and neuroinflammation	*In vivo*	[81]
22.	*Clivia miniata* bulbs, aerial parts and roots	Antioxidant, anti-Beta secretase, and anti-AChE	*In-vitro* and *in-silico*	[82]
23.	Arabian coffee and Date palm seed extract	Reduction of amyloid- beta; $A\beta_{42}$	*In vivo*	[83]
24.	Ethyl acetate fraction of *Cirsium japonicum*	inhibiting oxidative stress and $A\beta_{25-35}$ -induced AD	*In vivo*	[84]
25.	*Litsea cubeba* fruit powder	Inhibition of oxidative stress, decreased brain atrophy and Aβ plaques aggregation	*In vivo*	[85]
26.	*Hedyotis diffusa* N-butanol extract	Inhibition of Aβ mediated toxicity and oxidative stress	*In vivo*	[86]
27.	Raw and germinated black soybeans	Inhibition of cholinesterase and neuroinflammation	*In vivo*	[87]
28.	Polyphenols-rich extracts of *Desmodium elegans*	Anti-AChE and anti-BChE	*In vitro, in vivo and in silico*	[88]
29.	Ethanolic extract of *Diplazium esculentum* rich in phenolics	Beta secretase blocker, antioxidant and reduction of $A\beta_{42}$ peptides	*In vivo* and *in vitro*	[89]
30.	Extracts of *Hypericum perforatum*	Blocking of β-Amyloid Toxicity	*In vivo*	[90]
31.	Combination of Ginko biloba extract and docosahexaenoic acid	Improvement of memory and spatial learning, preservation of hippocampal structure and inhibition of neuroinflammation	*In vivo*	[91]
32.	Rice bran extract	Inhibition of neuroinflammation, Aβ42 deposition and p-tau protein accumulation	*In vitro*	[92]
33.	*Amaranthus dubius* aqueous leaf extract	Anticholinesterase and anti-oxidant activities	*In vivo*	[93]
34.	*Ginkgo biloba* extract	Inhibition of oxidative stress, DNA damage, mitochondria dysfunction and hippocampal neuronal damage	*In vivo*	[94]
35.	Blood Brain-Barrier-permeable aporphine-type alkaloids from *Nelumbo nucifera* flowers	Increases neurite outgrowth	*In vitro*	[95]
36.	Korean red ginseng derived from *Panax ginseng*	Inhibition of Aβ-Mediated oxidative stress, neuroinflammation and neuronal apoptosis	*In vitro*	[96]

No.	Name and nature of the plant extract	Activity	Model	References
37.	*Camellia sinensis* extracts	inhibit AChE activity	*In vitro*	[97]
38.	*Terminalia chebula* Retz. Extract	Inhibition of Aβ aggregation, Aβ-stimulated toxicity	*In vivo*	[98]
39.	Oxyresveratrol-β-cyclodextrin abundant in Mulberry tree	Anti-acetylcholinesterase and antioxidant activities	*In silico* and *in vivo*	[99]
40.	*Phoenix dactylifera* seed extract	Antioxidant, memory and behavior improvement	*In vivo*	[100]
41.	Components of *Hedyotis diffusa a*erial parts	Anti-cholinesterase and anti-beta secreatase	*In vitro*	[101]
42.	Aqueous and ethanolic extracts of *Cymbopogon citratus* leaf	Inhibition of oxidative stress, acetylcholinesterase and neuroinflammation	*In vivo*	[102]
43.	Ethanol extracts of *Allium subhirsutum* bulbs and aerial parts	Antioxidant and AChE inhibitory properties	*In vitro*	[103]
44.	*Morus nigra* fruit extract	Oxidative stress and Aβ-stimulated AD-like symptoms	*In vivo*	[104]
45.	Extracts of *Diplazium esculentum*	Antioxidants and Beta secretase inhibitors	*In vivo*	[105]

Table 1.
Plant-derived agents with preclinical anti-AD efficacy.

No	Name and nature of the plant extract	Activity	Study design	Duration	References
1.	Desalted *Salicornia europaea* alcohol extract	Frontal executive functioning among patients with Mild cognitive decline	Randomized, double-masked, placebo-controlled study	12 weeks	[112]
2.	Jiannao Yizhi preparation, a TCM formulation containing a combination of herbs	Improved blood levels of acetylcholine while reducing the amount of $A\beta_{42}$ and Tau in the serum among individuals suffering mild-moderate AD	Randomized, double-blind, clinical study	6 months	[113]
3.	Huannao yicong preparation, blend of herbs used in TCM	Reduction of blood levels of $A\beta_{42}$ and AChE with ultimate improvement of cognitive function among patients suffering mild-to-moderate AD	Randomized controlled double-blinded study	6 months	[114]
4.	Blend of β-Asarone present in *Acorus calamus*, tenuigenin from *Polygala tenuifolia* and memantine	Improved efficacy of memantine in management of moderate-to-severe AD	Non-randomized, single blinded study	12 weeks	[115]
5.	Yokukansan, a blend of seven herbs used in Kampo medicine	Improvement of symptoms; aggression/agitation and hallucinations among AD patients	Randomized double-masked placebo-controlled multisite study	4-weeks	[116]

No	Name and nature of the plant extract	Activity	Study design	Duration	References
6.	Davaie Loban used in Herbal medicine in Persian and Unani traditional medicine.	Memory improvement among patients suffering mild-moderate AD	Randomized double-masked placebo-controlled study	12 weeks	[110]
7.	Yishen Huazhuo, a TCM herbal formulation	Cognitive improvement among patients experiencing mild AD	Randomized controlled clinical trial	24 weeks	[117]
8.	Ninjin'yoeito (a formulation in traditional Japanese herbal medicine) combined with donepezil	Mild-to-moderate AD Cognitive improvement and reduction of AD-associated depression	Non-randomized, open-label prospective clinical trial	2 years	[118]

Table 2.
Plant-derived agents with clinical anti-AD efficacy.

and improved verbal memory deficits among the elderly with mild AD-like cognitive impairment in a 12-week clinical trial [108]. Guilingji, a formulation used in Traditional Chinese Medicine (TCM) containing 20 herbs demonstrated remarkable clinical efficacy in improving the quality of life and cognitive performance of AD patients during the 24 weeks of the study [109]. Davaie Loban herbal preparation was demonstrated to enhance memory among patients experiencing mild-to-moderate AD in a 12-week trial [110]. Dengzhan shengmai, a TCM formulation containing mainly *Erigeron breviscapus,* combined with donepezil hydrochloride was reported to improve quality of life, cognitive function and reduced neurotoxicity by decreasing levels of nitric oxide and endothelin among patients with AD [111]. Further, **Table 2** provides a summary of other herbal remedies which have provided efficacy against AD in clinical settings;

5. Conclusion

This chapter has briefly explored the possibilities of herbal preparations as alternatives for the management of AD. While at the moment there are limited options for management of AD, the opportunities afforded by medicinal plants offer a glimpse of hope in this fight. The progress in leveraging the prowess of medicinal plants as an alternative therapy for AD has been encouraging. The multifunctional nature of herbal preparations endows them with efficacy to tackle the complexity of AD pathophysiology. As demonstrated herein, AD pathology involves dysregulation of numerous key molecular pathways. Consequently, innovative drug design strategies for AD must actively pursue multifunctional therapeutic candidates, particularly herbal remedies. We believe that herbal-derived agents will play a fundamental role in overcoming the bottlenecks in the search for AD cure in the forthcoming future. We invite the reader to be on the lookout for this progress.

Conflict of interest

The authors declare no conflict of interest.

Author details

Daisy Jepkosgei Kipkemoi
University of South Australia, Adelaide, Australia

*Address all correspondence to: jepkosgeidaisy99@gmail.com

References

[1] Thakral S, Yadav A, Singh V, Kumar M, Kumar P, Narang R, et al. Alzheimer's disease: Molecular aspects and treatment opportunities using herbal drugs. Ageing Research Reviews. 2023;**88**:101960

[2] Alzheimer A, Stelzmann RA, Schnitzlein HN, Murtagh FR. An English translation of Alzheimer's 1907 paper, "Uber eine eigenartige Erkankung der Hirnrinde". Clinical Anatomy. 1995;**8**(6):429-431

[3] Barthélemy NR, Li Y, Joseph-Mathurin N, Gordon BA, Benzinger TLS, Buckles V, et al. Disease. Nature Medicine. 2020;**26**(3):398-407

[4] Korolev IO. Alzheimer's disease: A clinical and basic science review. Medical Student Research Journals. 2014;**4**(1):24-33

[5] Ding M, Qu Y, Hu B, An H. Biomedicine and pharmacotherapy signal pathways in the treatment of Alzheimer's disease with traditional Chinese medicine. Biomedicine and Pharmacotherapy. 2022;**152**:113208

[6] Rajasekhar K, Govindaraju T. Current progress, challenges and future prospects of diagnostic and therapeutic interventions in Alzheimer's disease. RSC Advances. 2018;**8**(42):23780-23804

[7] Scheltens P, Blennow K, Breteler MMB, De SB, Frisoni GB, Salloway S, et al. Alzheimer's disease. Lancet. 2016;**388**(10043):505-517

[8] Long S, Benoist C, Weidner W. World Alzheimer Report 2023: Reducing Dementia Risk: Never Too Early, Never Too Late. Alzheimer's Disease International: London, England; 2023

[9] Bush AI, Tanzi RE. Therapeutics for Alzheimer's disease based on the metal hypothesis. Neurotherapeutics. 2008;**5**(3):421-432

[10] Sharma K. Cholinesterase inhibitors as Alzheimer's therapeutics (review). Molecular Medicine Reports. 2019;**20**(2):1479-1487

[11] Syad AN, Devi KP. Botanics: A potential source of new therapies for Alzheimer's disease? Botanics: Targets and Therapy. 2014;**4**(2014):11-26

[12] Leung AY. Chinese Medicinals. In: Advances in New Crops. Portland, OR: Timber Press; 2011. pp. 499-510

[13] Flowers J. Koreans building a new world: Eastern medicine renaissance in the context of Japanese rule, 1910-1945 [doctoral dissertation]. Baltimore: Johns Hopkins University; 2019

[14] Najmi A, Javed SA, Al Bratty M, Alhazmi HA. Modern approaches in the discovery and development of plant-based natural products and their analogues as potential therapeutic agents. Molecules. 2022;**27**(2):349

[15] WHO. Traditional Medicine. 2024. Available from: https://www.afro.who.int/health-topics/traditional-medicine

[16] Srivastava A, Srivastava P, Pandey A, Khanna VK, Pant AB. Phytomedicine: A potential alternative medicine in controlling neurological disorders. In: New Look to Phytomedicine. Amsterdam: Elsevier Inc.; 2019. pp. 625-656

[17] Efferth T, Koch E. Complex interactions between phytochemicals. Therapeutic concept of phytotherapy.

Current Drug Targets. 2011;**12**(1): 122-132

[18] Bruno David JW, A DD. The pharmaceutical industry and natural products: Historical status and new trends. Phytochemistry Reviews. 2014;**14**:299-315

[19] Leonti M, Casu L. Traditional medicines and globalization: Current and future perspectives in ethnopharmacology. Frontiers in Pharmacology. 2013;**4**:1-13

[20] Malík M, Tlustoš P. Nootropic herbs, shrubs, and trees as potential cognitive enhancers. Plants. 2023;**12**(6):1364

[21] Patel J, King A, Malempati M, Patel M. Understanding nootropics and cognitive enhancement: Mechanism of action and ethical considerations. Health Open Research. 2024;**6**(2):1-13

[22] Suliman NA, Mat Taib CN, Mohd Moklas MA, Adenan MI, Hidayat Baharuldin MT, Basir R. Establishing natural nootropics: Recent molecular enhancement influenced by natural nootropic. Evidence-Based Complementary and Alternative Medicine. 2016;**2016**(1):1-112

[23] Tabassum N, Rasool S, Malik ZA, Ahmad F. Natural cognitive enhancers. Journal of Pharmacy Research. 2012;**5**(1): 153-160

[24] Kigen G, Kipkore W, Wanjohi B, Haruki B, Kemboi J. Medicinal plants used by traditional healers in Sangurur, Elgeyo Marakwet County, Kenya. Pharmacognosy Research. 2017;**9**(4):333-347

[25] Ratheesh G, Tian L, Reddy J. Role of medicinal plants in neurodegenerative diseases. Biomanufacturing Reviews. 2017;**2**(1):1-16

[26] Abdul Manap AS, Vijayabalan S, Madhavan P, Chia YY, Arya A, Wong EH, et al. *Bacopa monnieri*, a neuroprotective lead in Alzheimer disease: A review on its properties, mechanisms of action, and preclinical and clinical studies. Drug Target Insights. 2019;**13**:1-13

[27] Selkoe DJ, Hardy J. The amyloid hypothesis of Alzheimer's disease at 25 years. EMBO Molecular Medicine. 2016;**8**(6):595-608

[28] Sehar U, Rawat P, Reddy AP, Kopel J, Reddy PH. Amyloid beta in aging and Alzheimer's disease. International Journal of Molecular Sciences. 2022;**23**(21):12924

[29] Lacor PN, Buniel MC, Chang L, Fernandez SJ, Gong Y, Viola KL, et al. Synaptic targeting by Alzheimer's-related amyloid β oligomers. Journal of Neuroscience. 2004;**24**(45):10191-10200

[30] Kundo NK, Manik MI, Biswas K, Khatun R, Al-Amin MY, Alam AH, et al. Identification of polyphenolics from *Loranthus globosus* as potential inhibitors of cholinesterase and oxidative stress for Alzheimer's disease treatment. BioMed Research International. 2021;**2021**(1):1-16

[31] Ashrafian H, Hadi E, Hasan R. International journal of biological macromolecules review on Alzheimer's disease: Inhibition of amyloid beta and tau tangle formation. International Journal of Biological Macromolecules. 2021;**167**:382-394

[32] Grundke-Iqbal I, Iqbal K, Tung YC, Quinlan M, Wisniewski HM, Binder LI. Abnormal phosphorylation of the microtubule-associated protein tau (tau) in Alzheimer cytoskeletal pathology. National Academy of Sciences of the United States of America. 1986;**83**(13):4913-4917

[33] Rawat P, Sehar U, Bisht J, Selman A, Culberson J, Reddy PH. Phosphorylated tau in Alzheimer's disease and other tauopathies. International Journal of Molecular Sciences. 2022;**23**(21):12841

[34] Derry PJ, Hegde ML, Jackson GR, Kayed R, Tour JM, Tsai AL, et al. Revisiting the intersection of amyloid, pathologically modified tau and iron in Alzheimer's disease from a ferroptosis perspective. Progress in Neurobiology. 2020;**184**:101716

[35] Shukla V, Mishra SK, Pant HC. Oxidative stress in neurodegeneration. Advances in Pharmacological and Pharmaceutical Sciences. 2011;**2011**(1):572634

[36] Giacobini E, Gold G. Alzheimer disease therapy—Moving from amyloid-β to tau. Nature Reviews Neurology. 2013;**9**(12):677-686

[37] Luan K, Rosales JL, Lee K. Viewpoint: Crosstalks between neurofibrillary tangles and amyloid plaque formation. Ageing Research Reviews. 2013;**12**(1):174-181

[38] Babak SS, Alireza S, Mahnaz M. Amyloid-Beta: A crucial factor in Alzheimer's disease. Medical Principles and Practice. 2015;**24**(1):1-10

[39] Halder N, Lal G. Cholinergic system and its therapeutic importance in inflammation and autoimmunity. Frontiers in Immunology. 2021;**12**:660342

[40] Doyle CA, McDougle CJ. Cholinergic system. In: Volkmar FR, editor. Encyclopedia of Autism Spectrum Disorders. Cham: Springer; 2021. pp. 943-948

[41] Prado VF, Janickova H, Al-Onaizi MA, Prado MA. Cholinergic circuits in cognitive flexibility. Neuroscience. 2017;**345**:130-141

[42] Marucci G, Buccioni M, Dal Ben D, Lambertucci C, Volpini R, Amenta F. Efficacy of acetylcholinesterase inhibitors in Alzheimer's disease. Neuropharmacology. 2021;**190**:108352

[43] Martorana A, Esposito Z, Koch G. Beyond the cholinergic hypothesis: Do current drugs work in Alzheimer's disease? CNS Neuroscience & Therapeutics. 2010;**16**(4):235-245

[44] Huang Q, Liao C, Ge F, Ao J, Liu T. Acetylcholine bidirectionally regulates learning and memory. Journal of Neurorestoratology. 2022;**10**(2):100002

[45] Stanciu GD, Luca A, Rusu RN, Bild V, Beschea Chiriac SI, Solcan C, et al. Alzheimer's disease pharmacotherapy in relation to cholinergic system involvement. Biomolecules. 2019;**10**(1):40

[46] Pizzino G, Irrera N, Cucinotta M, Pallio G, Mannino F, Arcoraci V, et al. Oxidative stress: Harms and benefits for human health. Oxidative Medicine and Cellular Longevity. 2017;**2017**(1):8416763

[47] Lobo V, Patil A, Phatak A, Chandra N. Free radicals, antioxidants and functional foods: Impact on human health. Pharmacognosy Reviews. 2010;**4**(8):118

[48] Podsiedlik M, Markowicz-piasecka M. The influence of selected antipsychotic drugs on biochemical aspects of Alzheimer's disease. International Journal of Molecular Sciences. 2022;**23**(9):4621

[49] Picone P, Nuzzo D, Caruana L, Scafidi V, Di Carlo M. Mitochondrial dysfunction: Different routes to Alzheimer's disease therapy. Oxidative

Medicine and Cellular Longevity. 2014;**2014**(1):780179

[50] Singh A, Kukreti R, Saso L. Oxidative stress: A key modulator in neurodegenerative diseases. Molecules. 2019;**24**(8):1-20

[51] Li J, Wuliji, O, Li W, Jiang ZG, Ghanbari HA. Oxidative stress and neurodegenerative disorders. International Journal of Molecular Sciences. 2013;**14**(12):24438-24475

[52] Ezeani M, Omabe M. A new perspective of lysosomal cation channel-dependent homeostasis in Alzheimer's disease. Molecular Neurobiology. 2016;**53**:1672-1678

[53] Pritam P, Deka R, Bhardwaj A, Srivastava R, Kumar D, Jha AK, et al. Antioxidants in Alzheimer's disease: Current therapeutic significance and future prospects. Biology (Basel). 2022;**11**(2):212

[54] de Torre MP, Cavero RY, Calvo MI. Anticholinesterase activity of selected medicinal plants from Navarra region of Spain and a detailed phytochemical. Molecules. 2022;**27**(20):1-25

[55] Peng Y, Zhou C. Network pharmacology and molecular docking identify the potential mechanism and therapeutic role of *Scutellaria baicalensis* in Alzheimer's disease. Drug Design, Development and Therapy. 2024;**18**(2024):1199-1219

[56] Cao Q, Liu J, Dong P, Han H. Different ratios of *Schisandra chinensis* and *Evodia rutaecarpa* combination for treating Alzheimer's disease. Experimental Biology and Medicine. 2023;**248**(20):1877-1886

[57] Li H, Zheng T, Lian F, Xu T, Yin W, Jiang Y. Anthocyanin-rich blueberry extracts and anthocyanin metabolite protocatechuic acid promote autophagy-lysosomal pathway and alleviate neurons damage in vivo and in vitro models of Alzheimer's disease. Nutrition. 2021;**93**(2022):1-21

[58] Mooko T, Bala A, Tripathy S, Kumar CS, Mahadevappa CP, Chaudhary SK, et al. *Cannabis sativa* L. flower and bud extracts inhibited in vitro cholinesterases and β-secretase enzymes activities: Possible mechanisms of cannabis use in alzheimer disease. Endocrine, Metabolic and Immune Disorders-Drug Targets (Formerly Current Drug Targets-Immune, Endocrine and Metabolic Disorders). 2022;**22**(3):297-309

[59] Raghuvanshi R, Nuthakki VK, Singh L, Singh B. Phytomedicine identification of plant-based multitargeted leads for Alzheimer's disease: In-vitro and in-vivo validation of *Woodfordia fruticosa* (L.) Kurz. Phytomedicine. 2021;**91**:153659

[60] Yano M, Nakashima S, Kasa S, Nakamura S, Nishimura K, Oda Y, et al. Accelerative effects of carbazole-type alkaloids from *Murraya koenigii* on neurite outgrowth and their derivative's in vivo study for spatial memory. Journal of Natural Medicines. 2020;**74**:448-455

[61] Elhawary EA, Nilofar N, Zengin G, Eldahshan OA. Variation of the essential oil components of Citrus aurantium leaves upon using different distillation techniques and evaluation of their antioxidant, antidiabetic, and neuroprotective effect against Alzheimer's disease. BMC Complementary Medicine and Therapies. 2024;**24**(1):1-10

[62] Jara-Moreno D, Riveros AL, Barriga A, Kogan MJ, Delporte C. Inhibition of β-amyloid aggregation

of *Ugni molinae* extracts. Current Pharmaceutical Design. 2020;**26**(12):1365-1376

[63] Abu-Elfotuh K, Hamdan AM, Mohamed SA, Bakr RO, Ahmed AH, Atwa AM, et al. The potential anti-Alzheimer's activity of *Oxalis corniculata Linn*. Methanolic extract in experimental rats: Role of APOE4/LRP1, TLR4/NF-κβ/NLRP3, Wnt 3/β-catenin/GSK-3β, autophagy and apoptotic cues. Journal of Ethnopharmacology. 2024;**324**:117731

[64] Zeng P, Wang XM, Ye CY, Su HF, Tian Q. The main alkaloids in *Uncaria rhynchophylla* and their anti-Alzheimer's disease mechanism determined by a network pharmacology approach. International Journal of Molecular Sciences. 2021;**22**(7):3612

[65] Ono K, Zhao D, Wu Q, Simon J, Wang J, Radu A, et al. Pine bark polyphenolic extract attenuates amyloid-β and tau misfolding in a model system of Alzheimer's disease neuropathology. Journal of Alzheimer's Disease. 2021;**73**(4):1597-1606

[66] Liu D, Du D. Mulberry fruit extract alleviates cognitive impairment by promoting the clearance of amyloid-β and inhibiting neuroinflammation in Alzheimer's disease mice. Neurochemical Research. 2020;**45**(9):2009-2019

[67] Oboh G, Adedayo BC, Adetola MB, Oboh G, Christiana B, Blessing M, et al. Characterization and neuroprotective properties of alkaloid extract of *Vernonia amygdalina* Delile in experimental models of Alzheimer's disease characterization and neuroprotective properties of alkaloid extract of *Vernonia amygdalina* Delile in experimental models of Alzheimer's disease. Drug and Chemical Toxicology. 2020;**0**(0):1-10

[68] ALNasser MN, Mellor IR, Carter WG. A preliminary assessment of the nutraceutical potential of acai berry (Euterpe sp.) as a potential natural treatment for Alzheimer's disease. Molecules. 2022;**27**(15):4891

[69] Tan MA, Ishikawa H, An SSA. Pandanus amaryllifolius exhibits in vitro anti-amyloidogenic activity and promotes neuroprotective effects in amyloid-β-induced SH-SY5Y cells. Nutrients. 2022;**14**(19):3962

[70] Mohamed HE, Asker ME, Shaheen MA, Eissa RG, Younis NN. Alleviation of fructose-induced Alzheimer's disease in rats by pioglitazone and decaffeinated green coffee bean extract. Journal of Food Biochemistry. 2021;**45**(5):1-12

[71] Rehman S, Ali Ashfaq U, Sufyan M, Shahid I, Ijaz B, Hussain M. The insight of In Silico and In vitro evaluation of Beta vulgaris phytochemicals against Alzheimer's disease targeting acetylcholinesterase. PLoS One. 2022;**17**(3):0264074

[72] Boubakri A, Leri M, Bucciantini M, Najjaa H, Ben Arfa A, Stefani M, et al. Extract inhibits amyloid beta aggregation and toxicity involved in Alzheimer's disease. PLoS One. 2020;**15**(9):1-16

[73] Kwon OY, Lee SH. Ameliorating activity of *Ishige okamurae* on the amyloid Beta–induced cognitive deficits and neurotoxicity through regulating ERK, p38 MAPK, and JNK Signaling in Alzheimer's disease–like mice model. Molecular Nutrition & Food Research. 2020;**64**(12):1901220

[74] Gu L, Lu J, Li Q, Wu N, Zhang L, Li H, et al. A network-based analysis of key pharmacological pathways of *Andrographis paniculata* acting on

Alzheimer's disease and experimental validation. Journal of Ethnopharmacology. 2020;**251**(182):112488

[75] Temviriyanukul P, Sritalahareuthai V, Promyos N, Thangsiri S, Pruesapan K, Srinuanchai W, et al. The effect of sacred lotus (*Nelumbo nucifera*) and its mixtures on phenolic profiles, antioxidant activities, and inhibitions of the key enzymes relevant to Alzheimer's disease. Molecules. 2020;**25**(16):3713

[76] Kim DS, Zhang T, Park S. Protective effects of *Forsythiae fructus* and *Cassiae semen* water extract against memory deficits through the gut-microbiome-brain axis in an Alzheimer's disease model. Pharmaceutical Biology. 2022;**60**(1):212-224

[77] Sánchez-Martínez JD, Cifuentes A, Valdés A. Omics approaches to investigate the neuroprotective capacity of a *Citrus sinensis* (sweet orange) extract in a *Caenorhabditis elegans* Alzheimer's model. Food Research International. 2023;**172**:113128

[78] Ramasamy A, Anandakumar K, Kathiresan K. In-vitro antioxidant potential and acetylcholinesterase inhibitory effect of Ficus benghalensis aerial root extract. African Health Sciences. 2022;**22**(4):291-299

[79] Cheng D, Su L, Wang X, Li X, Li L, Hu M, et al. Extract of *Cynomorium songaricum* ameliorates mitochondrial ultrastructure impairments and dysfunction in two different in vitro models of Alzheimer's disease. BMC Complementary Medicine and Therapies. 2021;**21**(1):206

[80] Sharma H, Kim DY, Shim KH, Sharma N, An SS. Multi-targeting neuroprotective effects of Syzygium aromaticum bud extracts and their key phytocompounds against neurodegenerative diseases. International Journal of Molecular Sciences. 2023;**24**(9):8148

[81] Nam Y, Ji YJ, Shin SJ, Park HH, Yeon SH, Kim SY, et al. Platycodon grandiflorum root extract inhibits Aβ deposition by breaking the vicious circle linking oxidative stress and neuroinflammation in Alzheimer's disease. Biomedicine and Pharmacotherapy. 2024;**177**:117090

[82] Elnagar AS, Mohyeldin MM, Mostafa NM, Salaheldin S, Ibrahim A, Batiha GE, et al. Biomedicine & Pharmacotherapy Antioxidant and anti-Alzheimer activities of *Clivia miniata* (Lindl) roots, bulbs, and aerial parts: In-vitro and in-silico studies. Biomedicine and Pharmacotherapy. 2023;**167**:115382

[83] Zidan NS, Omran AME, Rezk SM, Atteia HH, Sakran MI. Anti- Alzheimer's disease potential of Arabian coffee versus date palm seed extract in male rats. Journal of Food Biochemistry. 2021;**46**(1):1-9

[84] Pang QQ, Kim JH, Choi JM, Song JL, Lee S, Cho EJ, et al. Maackii improves cognitive impairment under amyloid Beta25-35-induced Alzheimer's disease model. BioMed Research International. 2022;**2022**(1):4513998

[85] Lee K, Chu C, Chiang S. Ameliorating effect on Aβ-induced Alzheimer's mice by *Litsea cubeba* Persoon powder. Molecules. 2021;**26**(18):1-18

[86] Danqing L, Yujie G, Chengpeng Z, Hong Y, BiSheng H, Yan C. N-butanol extract of Hedyotis diffusa protects transgenic *Caenorhabditis elegans* from Aβ-induced toxicity. Phytotherapy Research. 2020;**35**(2):1048-1061

[87] Shabbir U, Tyagi A, Ham HJ, Deog-hwan O. Comprehensive profiling of bioactive compounds in germinated black soybeans via UHPLC-ESI-QTOF-MS/MS and their anti-Alzheimer's activity. PLoS One. 2022;**17**(1):1-17

[88] Mahnashi MH, Ashraf M, Hassan A, Ullah H, Zeb A, Ghufran M, et al. Biomedicine and pharmacotherapy polyphenol-enriched *Desmodium elegans* DC. Ameliorate scopolamine-induced amnesia in animal model of Alzheimer's disease: In vitro, In vivo and In Silico approaches. Biomedicine and Pharmacotherapy. 2023;**165**:115144

[89] Kunkeaw T, Suttisansanee U, Trachootham D, Karinchai J, Chantong B, Potikanond S, et al. *Diplazium esculentum* (Retz.) Sw. Reduces BACE-1 activities and amyloid peptides accumulation in drosophila models of Alzheimer's disease. Scientific Reports. 2021;**11**(1):23796

[90] El Menuawy A, Brüning T, Eiriz I, Hähnel U, Marthe F, Möhle L, et al. Apolar extracts of St. John's Wort alleviate the effects of β-amyloid toxicity in early Alzheimer's disease. International Journal of Molecular Sciences. 2024;**25**(2):1301

[91] Abdelmeguid NE, Khalil MI, Elhabet R, Sultan AS, Salam SA. Combination of docosahexaenoic acid and *Ginko biloba* extract improves cognitive function and hippocampal tissue damages in a mouse model of Alzheimer's disease. Journal of Chemical Neuroanatomy. 2021;**116**:101995

[92] Saad S, Din E, Abd S, Laila E, Salwa R, Basma F, et al. Possible role of rice bran extract in microglial modulation through PPAR—Gamma receptors in alzheimer's disease mice model. Metabolic Brain Disease. 2021;**36**(7):1903

[93] Kipkemoi DJ, Ireri AM, Ngugi MP. Cognition enhancing potential of aqueous leaf extract of *Amaranthus dubius* in mice. Journal of Evidence-Based Integrative Medicine. 2023;**28**:2515690X231211661

[94] Xia C, Zhou M, Dong X, Zhao Y, Jiang M, Zhu G, et al. Ginkgo biloba extract inhibits hippocampal neuronal injury caused by mitochondrial oxidative stress in a rat model of Alzheimer's disease. PLoS One. 2024;**19**(8):1-17

[95] Yano M, Nakashima S, Oda Y, Nakamura S, Matsuda H. BBB-permeable aporphine-type alkaloids in Nelumbo nucifera flowers with accelerative effects on neurite outgrowth in PC-12 cells. Journal of Natural Medicines. 2020;**74**:212-218

[96] Choi S, Lim JW, Kim H. Korean red ginseng inhibits amyloid-β-induced apoptosis and nucling expression in human neuronal cells. Pharmacology. 2020;**105**(9-10):586-597

[97] Baranowska-Wójcik E, Szwajgier D, Winiarska-Mieczan A. Regardless of the brewing conditions, various types of tea are a source of acetylcholinesterase inhibitors. Nutrients. 2020;**12**(3):709

[98] Zhao L, Duan Z, Wang Y, Wang M, Liu Y, Wang X, et al. Protective effect of *Terminalia chebula* Retz. Extract against A β aggregation and A β -induced toxicity in *Caenorhabditis elegans*. Journal of Ethnopharmacology. 2021;**268**:113640

[99] Agarwal T, Manandhar S, Famurewa AC, Gurram PC, Suggala RS, Sankhe R, et al. Oxyresveratrol-β-cyclodextrin mitigates streptozotocin-induced Alzheimer's model cognitive impairment, histone deacetylase activity in rats: in silico and in vivo studies. Scientific Reports. 2024;**14**(1):9897

[100] Ismail H, Khalid D, Ayub SB, Ijaz MU, Akram S, Bhatti MZ, et al. Effects of Phoenix dactylifera against streptozotocin-aluminium chloride induced Alzheimer's rats and their In Silico study. BioMed Research International. 2023;**2023**(1):1725638

[101] Park JH, Whang WK. Bioassay-guided isolation of anti-Alzheimer active components from the aerial parts of Hedyotis diff Usa and simultaneous analysis for marker compounds. Molecules. 2020;**25**(24):5867

[102] Madi YF, Choucry MA, El-marasy SA, Meselhy MR, El-kashoury EA. UPLC-Orbitrap HRMS metabolic profiling of *Cymbopogon citratus* cultivated in Egypt; neuroprotective effect against AlCl 3-induced neurotoxicity in rats. Journal of Ethnopharmacology. 2020;**259**:112930

[103] Sut S, Maggi F, Bruno S, Badalamenti N, Quassinti L, Bramucci M, et al. Hairy garlic (*Allium subhirsutum*) from Sicily (Italy): LC-DAD-MSn analysis of secondary metabolites and in vitro biological properties. Molecules. 2020;**25**(12):1-14

[104] Wang E, Wang N, Zou Y, Fahim M, Zhou Y, Yang H, et al. Black mulberry (*Morus nigra*) fruit extract alleviated AD-like symptoms induced by toxic Aβ protein in transgenic *Caenorhabditis elegans* via insulin DAF-16 signaling pathway. Food Research International. 2022;**160**(2022):1-15

[105] Kongsung S, Inthachat W, Chantong B, Suttisansanee U, On-Nom N, Chupeerach C, et al. Box–behnken design-based optimization of phytochemical extraction from *Diplazium esculentum* (Retz.) Sw. Associated with its antioxidant and anti-Alzheimer's properties. Molecules. 2024;**29**(10):2204

[106] Noguchi-shinohara M, Hamaguchi T, Iwasa K, Horimoto M, Yamada M, Ono K, et al. Effects of Melissa officinalis extract containing rosmarinic acid on cognition in older adults without dementia: A randomized controlled trial. Journal of Alzheimer's Disease. 2020;**91**(199):805-814

[107] Foroumandi E, Javan R, Moayed L, Fahimi H, Kheirabadi F, Neamatshahi M, et al. The effects of fenugreek seed extract supplementation in patients with Alzheimer's disease: A randomized, double-blind, placebo-controlled trial. Phytotherapy Research. 2023;**37**(1):285-294

[108] Jung SJ, Jung ES, Ha KC, Baek HI, Park YK, Han SK, et al. Efficacy and safety of sesame oil cake extract on memory function improvement: A 12-week, randomized, double-blind, placebo-controlled pilot study. Nutrients. 2021;**13**(8):2606

[109] Ming ZH, Yimiao LU, Huichan WA, Yu CA, Lina MA, Hui PE, et al. Guilingji capsule (龟龄集胶囊) for Alzheimer's disease: Secondary analysis of a randomized non-inferiority-controlled trial. Journal of Traditional Chinese Medicine. 2023;**43**(5):1019-1025

[110] Tajadini H, Saifadini R, Choopani R, Mehrabani M. Complementary therapies in medicine herbal medicine Davaie Loban in mild to moderate Alzheimer's disease: A 12-week randomized double-blind placebo-controlled clinical trial. Complementary Therapies in Medicine. 2015;**23**(6):767-772

[111] Huang P, He X-Y, Xu M. Dengzhan shengmai capsule combined with donepezil hydrochloride in the treatment of Alzheimer's disease: Preliminary findings, randomized and controlled clinical trial clinical information.

Revista da Associação Médica Brasileira. 2021;**67**(2):190-194

[112] Lee WJ, Shin YW, Kim DE, Kweon MH, Kim M. Effect of desalted *Salicornia europaea* L. ethanol extract (PM-EE) on the subjects complaining memory dysfunction without dementia: A 12 week, randomized, double-blind, placebo-controlled clinical trial. Scientific Reports. 2020;**10**(1):1-12

[113] Wang HC, Liu NY, Zhang S, Yang Y, Wang ZY, Wei Y, et al. Clinical experience in treatment of Alzheimer's disease with Jiannao Yizhi formula (健脑益智方) and routine western medicine. Chinese Journal of Integrative Medicine. 2020;**26**(3):212-218

[114] Yang Y, Liu JP, Fang JY, Wang HC, Wei Y, Cao Y, et al. Effect and safety of Huannao Yicong formula (还脑益聪方) on patients with mild-to-moderate Alzheimer's disease_ A randomized, double-blinded, donepezil-controlled trial (Chinese journal of integrative medicine) (2018). Chinese Journal of Integrative Medicine. 2019;**25**:574-581

[115] Chang W, Teng2 J. Combined application of tenuigenin and β -asarone improved the efficacy of memantine in treating moderate-to-severe Alzheimer's disease. Drug Design, Development and Therapy. 2018;**12**:455-462

[116] Furukawa K, Tomita N, Uematsu D, Okahara K, Shimada H, Ikeda M, et al. Randomized double-blind placebo-controlled multicenter trial of Yokukansan for neuropsychiatric symptoms in Alzheimer's disease. Geriatrics and Gerontology International. 2017;**17**(2):211-218

[117] Zhang Y, Lin C, Zhang L, Cui Y, Gu Y, Guo J, et al. Cognitive improvement during treatment for mild Alzheimer's disease with a Chinese herbal formula: A randomized controlled. PLoS One. 2015;**10**(6):1-14

[118] Kudoh C, Arita R, Honda M, Kishi T, Komatsu Y. Effect of ninjin'yoeito, a Kampo (traditional Japanese) medicine, on cognitive impairment and depression in patients with Alzheimer's disease: 2 years of observation. Psychogeriatrics. 2016;**16**(2):85-92

Section 4

Special Cases in Alternative Medicine

Chapter 7

Graphite Plate for Pervaporation Wound Therapy

Francis Omujal and Joseph Mukisa

Abstract

Graphitized carbon black is one of the carbon adsorbent biomaterials claimed to treat venomous wounds, but its efficacy has been debated by scientists. We have endeavored to explain the principle of the black stone as a graphite plate in wound therapy. The graphite plate is prepared using cattle and fish bones by pyrolysis. It has the ability to create vapor-pressure difference and promote toxin dehydration in the wound. In the process, bacterial membrane disruption and a reduction in reactive oxygen species production around the wound occurs. The permeant vapor decrease in the wound then reduces the swelling and bacterial infection on the wound surface, thus stimulating the growth of new tissue around the wound and vaporization of toxin. This promotes the secretion of growth factors that facilitate angiogenesis and extracellular matrix deposition in the wound, resulting in the release of cytokines for immune response regulation. The graphite plate can also affect the microenvironment around the wound including pH, temperature and reactive oxygen levels. Therefore, the graphite plate pervaporation is a promising and effective technique for the removal of trace amounts of organic material and infections introduced into the wound.

Keywords: graphite plate, pervaporation, wound therapy, infectious wounds, venomous wounds

1. Introduction

The skin is the largest organ of the human body, approximately 15% of adult body weight, and comprises three distinct layers: epidermis, dermis, and subcutaneous tissue [1]. Although the skin provides critical physiological functions to the body like protecting it against external factors, aiding in the retention of body fluids, and regulating body temperature, it is susceptible to damage that results in a wound. A wound is defined as an injury to the body due to violence, a bite, a sting, an accident, or surgery, or disease [2], and that injured part is vulnerable to bacterial infections. In medicine, wounds are classified as 'open' and 'closed' based on the underlying cause of their creation [3, 4]. An open wound is when the skin surface shows an open split or bruise, and the underlying tissues are exposed to the outside environment and experience bleeding. For instance, an open wound can be an incision, abrasion or superficial, gunshot, puncture or penetration. Open wounds are exposed to the external environment, which makes them vulnerable to infection [5]. On the basis of the physiology of the healing process, open wounds can be classified as acute and chronic. A wound is referred to as chronic when it has failed to heal for at least 6 weeks in an orderly and timely manner due to several reasons including infections, poor blood circulation, and underlying medical conditions like diabetes mellitus [2]. Closed wounds occur when the surface of injured skin remains intact while the underlying tissue gets damaged. For instance, closed wounds can be bruises, insect stings, and bites from poisonous insects or animals respectively. Closed wounds often show inflammation and pain, and the blood that escapes the blood system remains inside in the body tissue.

Treatment of wounds involves a complex pathophysiological process. It is estimated that wound management accounts for 2–3% of the overall healthcare expenses of a country [6, 7]. Therefore, efficient wound management is essential. While several wound management techniques have been developed, researchers are looking for better alternative solutions for wound healing. Of recent carbon materials have attracted attention of scientists as useful in infectious and venomous wound healing processes.

2. Skin-structured infectious wounds

There are several skin-structured infectious wounds among patients, and these include cellulitis, erysipelas, boils, abscesses, infected sores and sepsis.

2.1 Cellulitis

Cellulitis is a deep skin infection caused by bacteria, and it affects the limbs and around the eyes, mouth, the anus, or on the belly. When an injury occurs on the skin, resulting in a skin break, bacteria can enter the wound and cause an infection. Common symptoms of cellulitis include skin redness, skin swelling or inflammation, skin tenderness and warmness, pain, blistering or bruising around the swollen skin, fever, headache and chills, general body weakness, and red streaks from the original site of infection.

2.2 Erysipelas

Erysipelas is a variant of cellulitis caused by a toxin of *Streptococcus pyogenes*, occasionally streptococci of groups B, C, and D [8], that affect the dermis skin layer, though it may extend to the superficial cutaneous lymphatics. Erysipelas is characterized by a well-defined and raised area of redness affecting the lower extremities and the face.

2.3 Boils

A boil is an infection caused by *Staphylococcus aureus* bacteria that affect a hair follicle(s) and nearby skin tissues. The damage to the hair follicle can be caused by a hair fallout at the underlying skin tissues on the face, neck, armpit, buttocks, or thighs. Boils usually begin by showing a tender, pinkish-red, swollen, and firm area on the skin that later pains and fills with pus and dead tissue. Patients with boils can experience fever, fatigue, itching on part of the boil, and skin redness [9].

2.4 Abscesses

A skin abscess is a localized collection of pus that develops in response to an infection or to the presence of foreign material under the skin, for example, the armpit, inner thigh, the rectal area, the external vaginal area, on a finger or toe, knee, shoulder and foot. It appears as a painful, swollen area that is warm when touched. Abscesses are caused by either an inflammatory response to an infectious process caused by bacteria, parasite or any foreign substance within the body (e.g., a needle and nail splinter). It can also develop due to obstructed oil or sweat glands, inflammation of hair follicles on the body or scalp, or minor breaks and punctures of the skin or after a surgical procedure. In this case, the infectious organism or foreign material triggers an inflammatory response, which causes the body to form a cavity to contain the infectious agent and prevent it from spreading to other body parts. As a result, pus forms in that cavity due to dead cells, proteins, bacteria, and other dead debris. Patients with skin abscesses show symptoms of pain, compressible mass that is red, warm to the touch, and tender, and as it progresses, it may 'point' and come to a head with pustular drainage and spontaneous rapture. Abscess can also cause symptoms like fever, nausea, vomiting, and more skin redness.

2.5 Infected sores

An infected sore arises out of an invasion and multiplication of microorganisms (bacteria, parasites, etc.) on the skin. This may remain localized, or it may spread through the blood or lymphatic vessels. The presence of such microorganisms within the sore causes local tissue damage and impedes wound healing [10, 11]. Symptoms of wound infection include increasing pain, swelling and redness, fever, and sometimes nausea in more severe infections.

2.6 Sepsis

Sepsis is the most severe clinical form of infection in patients with infected wounds and develops when pathogens enter the lymphatic and blood vessels [12].

3. Envenomation

The wounds caused by a bite or sting can either be open or closed, but this type of wound results in the introduction of toxins into the wound, which directly interacts with body enzymes and cellular receptors around the tissue of the wound. These toxins are naturally occurring organic poison with toxic effects that range from minor to potentially fatal, even at extremely low doses [13]. Usually, toxins are produced by metabolic activities of living cells or organisms in animals and insects, and their chemical composition indicates a complex mixture of biogenic amines, lipids, nucleic acids, peptides, and proteins, for example in venoms [14]. Such wounds associated with venoms often show signs of pain, swelling, and sometimes progressive paralysis, nausea and vomiting, labored breathing, rapid heart rate, and blurred vision.

Venom is an animal-derived toxin, or zootoxin, that is actively delivered through a wound by means of a bite, sting, or similar action [15]. The venom is a complex mixture of biogenic amines, lipids, nucleic acids, peptides, and proteins (including enzymes) that act locally or systemically introduced to injure cells and tissues [14]. A wide variety of land and marine animals, including arthropods like spiders, centipedes, and scorpions; invertebrates like jellyfish, sea anemones, cone snails, and octopuses; fishes like stingrays, rockfishes, and toadfishes; amphibians like salamanders; reptiles like snakes, and lizards; mammals like shrews and bats can be responsible for causing venom wounds. The venoms contains 90% water, 10% proteins, and other trace elements. The proteolytic enzymes include arginine ester hydrolase, thrombin-like enzyme, collagenase, hyaluronidase A2(A), phospholipase B, phospholipase C, lactate dehydrogenase, phosphomonoesterase, phosphodiesterase, acetylcholinesterase, Ribonuclease (RNase), Deoxyribonuclease (DNase), 5-nucleotidase, nicotinamide dinucleotide (NAD+)-nucleotide and L-amino- acid oxidase. Envenomation severity may be classified into four grades: minimal, moderate, severe, and very severe [16]. Minimal envenomation has symptoms of mild pain, 15.0–22.5 cm edema, erythema, and no systemic symptoms. Moderate envenomation has symptoms of severe pain, tenderness, erythema, vomiting, petechiae, fever, weakness, 20–40 cm edema. Severe envenomation has symptoms of widespread pain, tenderness, ecchymosis, systemic signs, vertigo, 40–50 cm edema, and very severe rapid swelling, ecchymosis, central nervous system (CNS) symptoms, visual disturbance, shock, and convulsions. Symptoms of venom bites include puncture marks at the site of the bite; pain, rapid progressive swelling, sometimes with blistering, necrosis, and bruising; or mild to moderate local swelling with progressive paralysis. Patients can also experience nausea and vomiting, labored breathing, rapid heart rate, blurred vision, hypotension, shock, and coma.

4. Accidental injury

This an unintentional injury that happens to anyone out of human error, technological disaster, or other unforeseen circumstances, and causing damage to the skin, for example, falling, motor vehicle and other transportation accidents, industrial accidents, construction failures, and home accidents [17].

5. Wound treatment

Wound treatment is divided into five stages: hemostasis, inflammation, cellular migration and proliferation, protein synthesis and wound contraction, and remodeling [4, 18].

5.1 Hemostasis

Hemostasis happens once an injury occurs in the skin, and blood vessels undergo vasoconstriction to reduce blood flow and limit blood loss, resulting in tissue hypoxia and acidosis. At the hemostasis phase, the body takes immediate action to produce cytokines or clotting factors to stop bleeding, reduce blood loss, shorten the bleeding time, and reduce the blood volume. During clotting, blood cell proteins play an important role in the coagulation process. For example, fibrin can promote platelet aggregation, increase blood viscosity, and promote erythrocyte aggregation. The erythrocytes are covered with protein, forming a thick layer. The color of the dissolved blood that has clotted promotes blood coagulation quickly and effectively [19].

Production of cytokines, vasoconstriction, and platelet aggregation is the body's immediate response to injury to stop bleeding and happen in the first few minutes up to few hours. Timely and efficient hemostasis has a direct impact on patient survival rates. It provides a temporary barrier to protect the underlying tissues from further injury and infection [2]. Activated platelets secret various mediators, such as thromboxane A_2 and serotonin, which promote further platelet activation and vasoconstriction. The platelet plug serves as a provisional matrix for the subsequent stages of wound healing. Transforming growth factor β (TGF-β) promotes collagen matrix construction [2]. The highly interconnected porous structure, superior mechanical strength, good biocompatibility, and biodegradability are all necessary for the ideal hemostatic material with antimicrobial activity. The ability to promote tissue regeneration and cell proliferation is also considered to be the most valuable properties in the biomedical field [20].

5.2 Inflammation

During inflammation, cells are released to stop more damage, remove cellular debris and bacteria, and promote the formation of new blood vessels and extracellular components. Immune cells such as neutrophils and monocytes are recruited to the wound site and they release a variety of inflammatory mediators, including cytokines, chemokines, and growth factors, which play a vital role in activating immune cells, further attracting cells, and promoting healing [2]. Neutrophils, which usually reach peak concentration in the wound, 24h after injury, are responsible for phagocytosis, bacteria elimination, and cellular debris clearance from the wound bed. This can happen in the first 1–3 days.

5.3 Proliferation

During proliferation, granulation tissue, re-epitherization, and neovascularization take place in the wound. This can last between a few days up to a month. The proliferation phase of the healing cascade can initiate to restore the vascular network, form granulation tissue, deposit collagen, and re-epithelialize. This is crucial in providing nutrients and oxygen during wound healing. Angiogenesis, the process of new blood vessel formation, is triggered by the growth factors produced from platelets, such as vascular endothelial growth factor (VEGF), platelets derived growth factor (PDGF), basic fibroblast growth factor (bFGF), and the serine protease thrombin in the wound site. Fibroblasts are activated to increase as result of the growth factors released from the hemostatic clot, and then they will migrate from the nearby dermis to the wound. The production of collagen and fibronectin results in the formation of granulation tissue, which fills the wound gap [2].

5.4 Maturation and remodeling

At maturation and remodeling or scar formation, the wound achieves maximum strength and is completely healed. This may last between 1 and 3 years [21, 22]. The remodeling phase is the final stage of wound healing initiated at the end of granulation tissue development. During remodeling, fibroblasts undergo apoptosis, and the newly formed tissue optimizes its mechanical strength and function. Collagen synthesis and degradation then attain a gradual balance [3]. The rapid deposition of collagen III in the extracellular matrix is eventually substituted by the deposition of collagen I, which has greater tensile strength but takes longer to produce.

6. Use of graphite plate in wound healing

Graphitized carbon black from animal sources (sometimes referred to as 'black stone') is one of the carbon adsorbents that has been claimed to be used to treat infectious wounds and snake bites for centuries [23]. The black stone is often promoted more as a treatment for snakebite rather than first aid globally. The preparation of the black stone as graphite plate is done with bones from cattle and fish, using various techniques like pyrolysis, heat transfer, bio-catalysis, surface science, fluid mechanics, and biomechanics bioreactor design [24]. The bones are usually composed of water, organic material, and apatite [25]. The hydroxy apatite components, majorly calcium and phosphorus, with formula $Ca_{10}(PO_4)_6(OH)_2$ accounts for 93% [24]. When the bones are heated for a specific time and temperature, they produce calcined bones with a specific composition and structure: hydroxyapatite—$Ca_5(PO_4)_3(OH)_2$. The phosphates (PO_{43}) are partially replaced by carbonates (CO_3^{2-}), and some carbonates even occupy some of the hydroxyl (OH−) positions. The presence of hydroxyl groups in bone apatite plays a significant role in medicine, besides determining the crystalline structure, atomic order, and reactivity of the calcined bone. The pyrolysis process involves burning bones at 300–500°C to change color from cream to black and further raising the temperature to 600–700°C to change color to calcined white [26, 27]. Although water, carbon monoxide, hydrogen and carbon dioxide evaporate at less than 500°C [28], primary and secondary carbonates decomposition occurs forming a crystalline graphite [29]. The release of these gases also contributes to the formation of pores of different sizes in the plates [30]. The large organic protein molecules on the bones also degrade into smaller molecules of aromatic benzene rings [31], leading to the formation of a graphitic structure. The presence of nitrogen on the graphite is important for the arrangement of aromatic rings and graphitization [32]. Low carbon content, high surface area, high porosity, surface charge, pH, presence of functional groups, as well as nitrogen heteroatoms all combined create a novel catalytic support for the graphite plate [19, 33]. Bone graphitization affects the plate's behavior including its interactions with bacteria and toxins, making it suitable for pervaporation wound therapy.

7. Graphite plate in pervaporation wound therapy

Pervaporation is a membrane separation process where solute transport occurs through dense membranes [20, 25, 34, 35]. It can also be referred to as a low-energy alternative for distillation, which allows the separation of liquid mixtures, irrespective of their vapor-liquid equilibria [36]. The only difference between the two is that distillation is based on vapor pressure while pervaporation is predominantly interactions of the target molecules with the membrane material [37]. It is also important to note that the chemical nature and structure of membrane and solubility or sorption of the permeants are essential during pervaporation [38]. In recent decades, membrane technologies have attracted a lot of interest and great potential of exploitation in medicine [39]. In wound healing, oxygen is essential for the survival of cells involved in the wound healing process such as fibroblasts and endothelial cells, as it is needed to produce biological energy equivalents such as adenosine triphosphate (ATP). This energy plays a role in cellular processes and maintains normal cell functions like activation and migration of immune cells, collagen synthesis, skin tissue generation, and the formation of new blood vessels. Upon an injury, the wound experiences hypoxia, or a lack of oxygen, and this causes disrupted blood flow and increased demand for oxygen by the influx of inflammatory cells, which results in cellular damage and impaired function, thus obstructing tissue repair and recovery. This leads to the slow healing process and increased risk of infection. Moreover, there are more serious complications of dehydration occurring in the wound when low blood volume is supplied, thus causing a drop in blood pressure and the amount of oxygen in the body. The graphite plate causes pervaporation by creating a hemostatic sponge around the wound tissue with efficient antibacterial and good hemostatic ability [20]. In addition, the graphite plate has ability to cause flash (or partial) evaporation in the wound. The blood in the wound experiences a reduction in pressure when it passes through a graphite plate. Such saturated blood in the wound with toxins and richer in the more volatile components is flash vaporized. The multi-components toxins in the blood in the wound then undergo a simple distillation process.

7.1 Infectious wounds

Bacteria can damage tissue around the wound both by eliciting a robust antibacterial immune response and releasing toxins that act locally or systemically to injure cells [14]. Invading bacteria can release toxins into infected tissues, by ingestion of improperly preserved food, inhalation, of the main active components or incidental contaminants, and exposure to certain agents. Wound healing is a complex process that can be impaired by various factors such as chronic inflammation, bacterial infection, diseases, and hypoxia [2]. Bacteria infected wounds are usually embedded with polysaccharides, proteins, and nucleic acids, which form a matrix for biofilm around the wound [3]. However, complete removal of biofilms in the wound created by bacteria like *Pseudomonas aeruginosa* and methicillin-resistant *Staphylococcus aureus* can be achieved using a graphite plate by disrupting bacterial membranes and reducing Reactive Oxygen Species (ROS) production in the wound [40]. In addition, the graphite plate can promote the secretion of growth factors that facilitate angiogenesis and extracellular matrix deposition, plus promoting the release of cytokines for immune response regulation in the wound. The physical interactions of the graphite plate with bacteria results in membrane piercing, surface adhesion, wrapping, and lipid extraction, in addition to disrupting the redox reactions as in the biomolecules, such as proteins, lipids, and DNA [41]. In the process, the microenvironment around the wound like pH, temperature, and reactive oxygen levels are altered. The pH environment in the wound often varies depending on the stage of the wound. For instance, acute and chronic wounds have an acidic pH that ranges from 5.5 to 7.5 (normal skin pH is 4.5). Usually, the area around the wound often experiences increased temperature and reduced oxygen level. The graphite plate produces an optimum acidic pH that can prevent bacterial growth in the wound. For instance, it can create an alkaline pH that is suitable for healing chronic wounds [2]. It can also increase oxygen around the wound through pervaporation, which leads to an optimum pH and limits the production of reactive oxygen species (ROS) around the wound. Oxygen is a vital component in wound healing, especially in re-epithelialization, angiogenesis, and infection resistance. With low oxygen level in the wound, cells tend to increase the production of ROS to compensate for lack of oxygen, and excessive production ROS levels can lead to oxidative stress, cellular damage, and inflammation due to H_2O_2 production, thus impeding wound healing. The graphite plate can deliver oxygen to the wound. Enzymes in the mammalian blood and liver (e.g., catalase) are responsible for oxidizing diverse electron-donating substrates, resulting in H_2O_2 breakdown and O_2 production. The graphite plate acts as a ROS-scavenging antioxidant and increases the production of oxygen. The release of oxygen by the graphite plate will depend on the particle size and surface area of the plate, and the surrounding temperature and humidity around the wound. The graphite plate can also lead to an appropriate electrical stimulation around the wound that produces a range of effects like antibacterial properties, promotion of cell proliferation, and induction of angiogenesis. The electric field around the wound can cause cell proliferation and migration, leading to a healing effect.

7.2 Venomous wounds

In developing countries, if a person gets bitten by a venomous animal, arthropod, insect, and reptile, there is a tendency to seek treatment from a traditional health practitioner. A black stone is often the most common method for its treatment before seeking treatment in the nearest clinic or hospital, but its use has been debated among scientists and physicians for over a century. Therefore, it is better to explore the various modes of action of the black stone in the management of venomous wounds. The black stone as a graphite plate uses the variant of negative pressure wound therapy or vacuum-assisted closure principle. The graphite plate applies sub-atmospheric pressure (e.g., 40–200 mmHg) on the wound in order to reduce inflammation, exudate, and improve granulation tissue formation. This causes an increase in blood flow, reduces redness and swelling, and helps draw wound edges together, resulting in a healing effect. Sometimes, the wound healing approach is referred to as hemoperfusion, where blood undergoes filtration to remove possible toxins injected by a venomous animal.

The graphite plate applies the principle of pervaporation around the venomous wound. In this case, the graphite plate is directly plugged into a blood drop of the open wound, and toxins in the blood are separated by partial vaporization through a porous or nonporous membrane of the graphite plate. The assumption is that the process has an isothermal operation. There is plug and flow on the feed side of the plate while pressure drops around the wound with a perfect blood mix inflow in the wound, and steady flow operation. The diversity in the chemical composition of venom drives pervaporation process due to differences in their chemical potential concentration gradient between phases on the opposite sides of the plate. The nitrogen heteroatoms affixed to the graphite plate, effectively remove trace amounts of organic species that may have been introduced into the bloodstream. A small amount of latent heat from the bloodstream due to toxins in the wound can selectively permeate through the graphite plate.

The hydrophobicity of the graphite plate also prevents mass transfer of the blood in the wound by creating a vapor-liquid interface, and this causes the graphite plate to stick to the wound. In the process, blood is left intact but continues to flow normally, without any clotting factors, as the permeant vapor is swept away by gas on the downstream side of the plate, thus causing wound healing. Low temperatures and pressures around the wound are needed to efficiently transfer biological toxin vapor species contained in the blood from one side of the plate to the opposite side [42]. The method has also been found suitable for the treatment of boils and abscesses, infected wound sores, accident injuries, or bruises wounds.

8. Practical procedures of the graphite plate pervaporation wound therapy

8.1 Step one

- Create a feed stream for the graphite plate by opening up any closed wound using a sharp instrument like a needle or razorblade to release a blood drop(s). The bigger the blood drop or, the more blood drops you see before placing the plate, the faster the wound will heal.

- Place the plate on the blood drops and it immediately plug itself tight to the wound, stopping any bleeding.

- In an open wound where the edges have drawn apart, do not place the graphite plate on the exposed blood vessels and nerves, but open up the skin next to the edge of the wound or open up the skin at the center surrounded by the bite lacerations.

8.2 Step two

- Place the graphite plate on the blood drops and leave it there. The hydrophobic nature of the graphite plate prevents the mass transfer of the blood in the wound by creating a vapor-liquid interface, while the vapor-pressure difference triggered by temperature difference between the two bounding surfaces causes the graphite plate to stick on the wound.

- The permeant vapor from the blood is swept away by gas on the downstream side of the plate.

- Temperature and vapor are transferred from the bloodstream to the plate, lowering not only the body's temperature but also the partial pressure difference between the wound and the plate until equilibrium is reached and reactions stop, and then the plate will drop off.

- Allow the plate to stick for a few hours, a day or two, sometimes after a week, like in an infected sore. The pain ceases, inflammation disappears, and the wound gets completely healed.

Precautions

- For venom wounds or bite, it is highly recommended to use the graphite plate, especially in the first hour after the bite, before severe septic shock sets in.

- In boils, abscesses, and cellulitis, it is highly recommended to use the plate in the first 7 days, before tissues start to rot and degenerate into pus.

- It is not advisable to pluck the graphite plate from the wound and wait for it to detach itself.

- The patient is free to move about with the graphite plate and care should be taken not to interfere with the stuck graphite plate on the wound.

- A bandage, (not a sticking tape), plaster, string, cloth, or anything else, may be used to keep the graphite plate in place, especially when going to bed or when moving about.

- The graphite plate is hydrophobic in its nature and therefore avoid, making it wet when in use. In case the patient needs to bathe, let him or her use a wet napkin or towel.

9. Conclusion

The graphite plate effectively removes trace amounts of toxins introduced into the bloodstream by creating vapor-pressure differences triggered by temperature differences in the wound. The permeant vapor from the blood in the wound is removed as it promotes healing. Therefore, pervaporation wound therapy can be a new technology to be used in wound management.

Author details

Francis Omujal[1*] and Joseph Mukisa[2]

1 Natural Chemotherapeutics Research Institute, Ministry of Health, Uganda

2 Madstone Pharma Limited, Uganda

*Address all correspondence to: fomujal@gmail.com

References

[1] Kolarsick PA, Kolarsick MA, Goodwin C. Anatomy and physiology of the skin. Journal of the Dermatology Nurses' Association. 2011;**3**(4):203-213

[2] Han X, Ju LS, Irudayaraj J. Oxygenated wound dressings for hypoxia mitigation and enhanced wound healing. Molecular Pharmaceutics. 2023;**20**(7):3338-3355

[3] Ji S, Xiao S, Xia Z, Chinese Burn Association Tissue Repair of Burns and Trauma Committee, Cross-Straits Medicine Exchange Association of China. Consensus on the treatment of second-degree burn wounds. Burns & Trauma. 2024;**12**:tkad061

[4] Nethi SK, Das S, Patra CR, Mukherjee S. Recent advances in inorganic nanomaterials for wound-healing applications. Biomaterials Science. 2019;**7**(7):2652-2674

[5] Cao W, Peng S, Yao Y, Xie J, Li S, Tu C, et al. A nanofibrous membrane loaded with doxycycline and printed with conductive hydrogel strips promotes diabetic wound healing in vivo. Acta Biomaterialia. 2022;**152**:60-73

[6] Järbrink K, Ni G, Sönnergren H, Schmidtchen A, Pang C, Bajpai R, et al. The humanistic and economic burden of chronic wounds: A protocol for a systematic review. Systematic Reviews. 2017;**6**:1-7

[7] Sadat Z, Farrokhi-Hajiabad F, Lalebeigi F, Naderi N, Gorab MG, Cohan RA, et al. A comprehensive review on the applications of carbon-based nanostructures in wound healing: From antibacterial aspects to cell growth stimulation. Biomaterials Science. 2022;**10**(24):6911-6938

[8] Opriessnig T, Coutinho TA. Erysipelas. Diseases of Swine. 2019;**53**:835-843. DOI: 10.1002/9781119350927.ch53

[9] Bandi VUG. Holistic approach of homoeopathy in treatment of boils [doctoral dissertation]. India: Rajiv Gandhi University of Health Sciences; 2009

[10] López-Cortés A, Abarca E, Silva L, Velastegui E, León-Sosa A, Karolys G, et al. Identification of key proteins in the signaling crossroads between wound healing and cancer hallmark phenotypes. Scientific Reports. 2021;**11**(1):17245

[11] Scalise A, Bianchi A, Tartaglione C, Bolletta E, Pierangeli M, Torresetti M, et al. Microenvironment and microbiology of skin wounds: The role of bacterial biofilms and related factors. In Seminars in Vascular Surgery. Vol. 28, 3-4. Pennsylvania, United States: WB Saunders; 2015. pp. 151-159. DOI: 10.1053/j.semvascsurg.2016.01.003

[12] Taati Moghadam M, Khoshbayan A, Chegini Z, Farahani I, Shariati A. Bacteriophages, a new therapeutic solution for inhibiting multidrug-resistant bacteria causing wound infection: Lesson from animal models and clinical trials. Drug Design, Development and Therapy. 2020;**14**:1867-1883

[13] Gupta M, Naik AK, Singh SK. Bacteriological profile and antimicrobial resistance patterns of burn wound infections in a tertiary care hospital. Heliyon. 2019;**5**(12):1-4. DOI: 10.1016/j.heliyon.2019.e02956

[14] Bolon B, Heinz-Taheny K, Yeung KA, Oguni J, Erickson TB, Chai PR, et al.

Animal toxins. In: Haschek and Rousseaux's Handbook of Toxicologic Pathology. 3rd edition. Academic Press; 2023. pp. 547-628. DOI: 10.1016/C2010-1-67850-9

[15] Gupta R, Darby GC, Imagawa DK. Efficacy of negative pressure wound treatment in preventing surgical site infections after Whipple procedures. The American Surgeon. 2017;**83**(10):1166-1169

[16] Coppola CM, Hogan DE. When a snake bites. Journal of Osteopathic Medicine. 1994;**94**(6):494-494

[17] Scotti JR, Ruggiero KJ, Rabalais AE. The traumatic impact of motor vehicle accidents. In: La Greca AM, Silverman WK, Vernberg EM, Roberts MC, editors. Helping Children Cope with Disasters and Terrorism. American Psychological Association. APA PsycBooks; 2002. pp. 259-291. DOI: 10.1037/10454-012

[18] Ji W, Li B, Li N, Xing C. Design strategy of microneedle systems for skin wound healing: Based on the structure of tips and therapeutic methodologies. ACS Applied Bio Materials. 2024;**7**(7):4254-4269. DOI: 10.1021/acsabm.4c00532

[19] Liu D, Yang P, Gao M, Yu T, Shi Y, Zhang M, et al. NLRP3 activation induced by neutrophil extracellular traps sustains inflammatory response in the diabetic wound. Clinical Science. 2019;**133**(4):565-582

[20] Fang Y, Nie T, Li G, Wang L, Du J, Wu J. Multifunctional antibiotic hydrogel doped with antioxidative lycopene-based liposome for accelerative diabetic wound healing. Chemical Engineering Journal. 2024;**480**:147930

[21] Raziyeva K, Kim Y, Zharkinbekov Z, Kassymbek K, Jimi S, Saparov A. Immunology of acute and chronic wound healing. Biomolecules. 2021;**11**(5):700

[22] Wallace ER, Yue Z, Dottori M, Wood FM, Fear M, Wallace GG, et al. Point of care approaches to 3D bioprinting for wound healing applications. Progress in Biomedical Engineering. 2023;**5**(2):1-22. DOI: 10.1088/2516-1091/acceeb

[23] Omara T, Kagoya S, Openy A, Omute T, Ssebulime S, Kiplagat KM, et al. Antivenin plants used for treatment of snakebites in Uganda: Ethnobotanical reports and pharmacological evidences. Tropical Medicine and Health. 2020;**48**:1-16

[24] Said J, Walker M, Parsons D, Stapleton P, Beezer AE, Gaisford S. An in vitro test of the efficacy of an anti-biofilm wound dressing. International Journal of Pharmaceutics. 2014;**474**(1-2):177-181

[25] Snoeck C, Lee-Thorp JA, Schulting RJ. From bone to ash: Compositional and structural changes in burned modern and archaeological bone. Palaeogeography, Palaeoclimatology, Palaeoecology. 2014;**416**:55-68

[26] Afolabi YT. Catalytic performance of calcium oxide (cao) using calcined animal bones and waste cooking oils for trans-esterification [master's thesis]. Nigeria: Kwara State University; 2022

[27] Nicholson RA. A morphological investigation of burnt animal bone and an evaluation of its utility in archaeology. Journal of Archaeological Science. 1993;**20**(4):411-428

[28] Feng D, Zhao Y, Zhang Y, Sun S, Meng S, Guo Y, et al. Effects of K and Ca on reforming of model tar compounds with pyrolysis biochars under H_2O or CO_2. Chemical Engineering Journal. 2016;**306**:422-432

[29] Piccirillo C. Preparation, characterisation and applications of bone char, a food waste-derived sustainable material: A review. Journal of Environmental Management. 2023;**339**:117896

[30] Cortes H, Caballero-Florán IH, Mendoza-Muñoz N, Córdova-Villanueva EN, Escutia-Guadarrama L, Figueroa-González G, et al. Hyaluronic acid in wound dressings. Cellular and Molecular Biology. 2020;**66**(4):191-198

[31] Hu JC, Zheng CX, Sui BD, Liu WJ, Jin Y. Mesenchymal stem cell-derived exosomes: A novel and potential remedy for cutaneous wound healing and regeneration. World Journal of Stem Cells. 2022;**14**(5):318

[32] Muretta JE. Investigation of the Structure, Chemistry and Functional Performance of Novel Biochars. A dissertation submitted in partial fulfillment of the requirements for the degree of Doctor of Philosophy Montana Tech of the University of Montana, Butte, Unites States. 2022

[33] Tanaka S, Yasuda T, Katayama Y, Miyake Y. Pervaporation dehydration performance of microporous carbon membranes prepared from resorcinol/formaldehyde polymer. Journal of Membrane Science. 2011;**379**(1-2):52-59

[34] Figoli A, Santoro S, Galiano F, Basile A. Pervaporation membranes: Preparation, characterization, and application. In: Pervaporation, Vapour Permeation and Membrane Distillation. Sawston, United Kingdom: Woodhead Publishing; 2015. pp. 19-63

[35] Van der Bruggen B, Luis P. Pervaporation. In: Progress in Filtration and Separation. Cambridge, Massachusetts, United States: Academic Press; 2015. pp. 101-154. DOI: 10.1016/C2009-0-64471-8

[36] Essalhi M, Khayet M. Fundamentals of membrane distillation. In: Pervaporation, Vapour Permeation and Membrane Distillation. Sawston, United Kingdom: Woodhead Publishing; 2015. pp. 277-316

[37] Vandezande P. Next-generation pervaporation membranes: Recent trends, challenges and perspectives. In: Pervaporation, Vapour Permeation and Membrane Distillation. Sawston, United Kingdom: Woodhead Publishing; 2015. pp. 107-141

[38] Crespo JG, Brazinha C. Fundamentals of pervaporation. In: Pervaporation, Vapour Permeation and Membrane Distillation. Sawston, United Kingdom: Woodhead Publishing; 2015. pp. 3-17

[39] Galiano F, Castro-Muñoz R, Figoli A. Pervaporation, vapour permeation and membrane distillation: From membrane fabrication to application. Membranes. 2021;**11**(3):162

[40] Wang W, Cui Y, Wei X, Zang Y, Chen X, Cheng L, et al. $CuCo_2O_4$ nanoflowers with multiple enzyme activities for treating bacterium-infected wounds via Cuproptosis-like death. ACS Nano. 2024;**18**(24):15845-15863. DOI: 10.1021/acsnano.4c02825

[41] Zheng H, Ma R, Gao M, Tian X, Li YQ, Zeng L, et al. Antibacterial applications of graphene oxides: Structure-activity relationships, molecular initiating events and biosafety. Science Bulletin. 2018;**63**(2):133-142

[42] Bolto B, Hoang M, Gray SR, Xie Z. New generation vapour permeation membranes. In: Pervaporation, Vapour Permeation and Membrane Distillation. Sawston, United Kingdom: Woodhead Publishing; 2015. pp. 247-273

Chapter 8

An Ayurvedic Approach to Constipation

Shweta Parwe and Milind Nisargandha

Abstract

This chapter will express an Ayurvedic approach to constipation, a common digestive disease that affects millions of people around the world. Constipation is described as the inability to empty the intestines or the passage of hard stools. Constipation is caused by an imbalance of the vata dosha, which governs the movement and evacuation of waste particles from the body. The chilly, dry, harsh features of vata dosha disrupt and impair intestinal function. The chapter will go through Ayurvedic constipation solutions such as natural laxatives, dietary adjustments, exercise, massage, and lifestyle changes. Triphala, castor oil, psyllium husk, flax seeds, and raisins are some of the natural laxatives. Dietary changes include eating more fruits and vegetables, whole grains, and warm drinks while avoiding cold, dry, heavy, and processed foods. The abdominal muscles are stimulated and blood circulation to the digestive organs is improved by exercise and massage treatments. Changes in lifestyle modification follow a regular routine, avoiding stress, proper sleep, and practicing meditation for lifestyle improvements. The chapter will also go over the benefits of Ayurveda for constipation alleviation, such as improved digestion, increased immunity, prevention of problems, well-being, and how to apply the Ayurvedic approach to constipation in everyday life.

Keywords: Malavstambha, constipation, Ayurvedic intervention, digestion, elimination

1. Introduction

Constipation (Malavashtambha) is a frequent digestive problem (indigestion) that affects people of all age groups and has a bad impact on the digestive system which leads to negatives effect on their quality of life. Constipation is regarded in Ayurveda as a manifestation of an imbalance in the Vata dosha, which governs movement and elimination in the body. This chapter explores the Ayurvedic perspective on constipation (malavstambha), including its causes, symptoms, and the fundamental Ayurvedic principles that dictate its treatment. Understanding constipation through the lens of Ayurveda allows individuals to take a holistic and natural approach to alleviating this ailment and achieving overall wellness.

2. Ayurvedic concept of digestion and elimination

In the Ayurvedic concept Agni, is often referred to as the "digestive fire," and it is considered the cornerstone of good health and vitality. It represents the transformative and metabolic processes that occur within the body, especially in the context of digestion and assimilation of food. The concept of Agni is central to Ayurvedic medicine, as it plays a crucial role in determining the overall well-being of an individual.

Agni is not just a physical entity but also a subtle force that governs the transformation of food into nutrients, energy, and waste products. It is responsible for breaking down ingested food into its constituent elements, extracting essential nutrients, and eliminating waste materials efficiently. In Ayurvedic Panchakarma recognizes several types of Agni, each serving a specific function in the digestive process:

Jatharagni (Primary Digestive Fire): This is the main digestive fire located in the stomach and small intestine. It is responsible for the initial breakdown of food and the secretion of digestive enzymes, gastric juices, and bile.

Bhutagni (Elemental Digestive Fire): Bhutagni governs the transformation of specific elements within food. Each of the five elements (earth, water, fire, air, and ether) in the food is metabolized by its equivalent Bhutagni.

Dhatvagni (Tissue Digestive Fire): Dhatvagni operates at the cellular level, ensuring that the nutrients derived from food are absorbed and utilized by the body to nourish the various tissues and organs [1].

2.1 The role of Agni in the digestive process

Initiation of Digestion: When food is ingested, Agni is responsible for initiating the digestion process. It signals the release of digestive juices, enzymes, and hydrochloric acid in the stomach, which begin to break down the food and make it chyame.

Transformation of Food: Agni converts the ingested food into simpler and absorbable forms. Carbohydrates are broken down into sugars l.e Glucose, proteins into amino acids, and fats into fatty acids and glycerol.

Absorption of Nutrients: Agni ensures the proper absorption of nutrients from the broken-down food. Nutrients are absorbed through the intestinal walls into the bloodstream to be transported to various tissues and organs.

Elimination of Waste: After extracting the necessary nutrients, Agni facilitates the elimination of waste materials and toxins from the body through the process of excretion. This helps maintain a clean and healthy gastrointestinal tract (GIT).

2.2 Signs of balanced Agni

Regular and comfortable bowel movements Absence of bloating, gas, or indigestion Strong appetite and efficient digestion Clear and radiant skin Sustained energy levels and mental clarity Signs of Imbalanced Agni:

Irregular or sluggish bowel movements Bloating, gas, or indigestion Lack of appetite or excessive hunger Fatigue, lethargy, and mental fog Accumulation of toxins (Ama) in the body Promoting Balanced Agni:

In Ayurveda Panchakarma emphasizes the importance of maintaining balanced Agni for overall health. Several factors can influence Agni, including diet, lifestyle, emotional state, and environmental conditions. To promote balanced Agni, we have to follow the Ayurvedic guidelines including:

Eating mindfully and in a calm environment Consuming freshly cooked, warm, and nourishing foods Avoiding overeating or consuming heavy, difficult-to-digest foods Incorporating digestive spices like ginger, cumin, and fennel into meals. Following a regular daily routine, including consistent meal timings and Managing stress through practices like meditation and relaxation techniques By nurturing the Agni, individuals can improve their digestive health, enhance nutrient absorption, and experience increased vitality and overall well-being.

The significance of balanced Agni for smooth and regular bowel movements is profound in Ayurveda. Agni, the digestive fire, is responsible for breaking down ingested food, extracting nutrients, and eliminating waste products efficiently. When Agni is balanced, the entire digestive process functions smoothly, leading to regular bowel movements and optimal gastrointestinal health. Here are some key aspects highlighting the importance of balanced Agni for smooth and regular bowel movements:

Efficient Digestion: Balanced Agni ensures the efficient digestion of food. It breaks down complex nutrients into simpler forms that are easily absorbed and assimilated by the body. This prevents the accumulation of undigested food particles that can lead to constipation and other digestive issues.

Proper Nutrient Absorption: When Agni is balanced, it facilitates the proper absorption of nutrients from the digested food. Adequate absorption of nutrients is essential for nourishing the body and supporting various bodily functions, including muscle function and cellular repair.

Elimination of Waste: Balanced Agni promotes the timely elimination of waste materials and toxins from the body. It prevents the accumulation of Ama (undigested waste) in the digestive tract, which can disrupt bowel movements and lead to constipation (malavashtambha).

Maintenance of Gut Flora: A balanced Agni supports a healthy gut microbiome. The gut flora plays a crucial role in digestion, and a harmonious balance of beneficial microorganisms helps maintain smooth bowel movements and regularity.

Prevention of Constipation: Constipation often results from slow or inefficient digestion, leading to the inadequate movement of stool through the intestines. Balanced Agni ensures that the digestive process is neither too sluggish nor too rapid, thus preventing constipation.

Prevention of Diarrhea: On the other hand, excessive or imbalanced Agni can lead to diarrhea, as food may pass through the digestive tract too quickly, leaving little time for proper nutrient absorption and water reabsorption.

Reduction of Gas and Bloating: Balanced Agni helps prevent the accumulation of undigested food, which can lead to gas and bloating. Proper digestion and assimilation reduce the likelihood of these discomforts.

Enhanced Peristalsis: Peristalsis is the rhythmic contraction and relaxation of the intestinal muscles that propel stool through the digestive tract. Balanced Agni supports regular and coordinated peristaltic movements, promoting smooth bowel movements.

2.3 Ayurvedic approach to balancing Agni for smooth bowel movements

Mindful Eating: Eating calmly and mindfully allows the body to focus on the digestive process fully.

Balanced Diet: Consuming a balanced diet that includes easily digestible foods and a variety of nutrients supports balanced Agni.

Adequate Hydration: Proper hydration helps in the softening of stool, making bowel movements more comfortable and regular.

Herbal Support: Ayurvedic herbs like ginger, cumin, and Triphala are known to support balanced Agni and promote regular bowel movements.

Avoiding Overeating: Overeating can overload the digestive system, leading to sluggish digestion and constipation.

Stress Management: Chronic stress can negatively impact Agni. Managing stress through relaxation techniques can support digestive health.

In conclusion, balanced Agni is crucial for smooth and regular bowel movements. Ayurvedic principles emphasize the significance of nurturing Agni to promote optimal digestion, assimilation of nutrients, and timely elimination of waste, ultimately supporting overall gastrointestinal health.

In Ayurveda, the gastrointestinal tract is viewed as a critical system responsible for the digestion and assimilation of food. It plays a central role in maintaining overall health and well-being. According to Ayurveda, the gastrointestinal tract is influenced by the three doshas - Vata, Pitta, and Kapha - which govern various physiological functions. The balance of these doshas is essential for maintaining digestive health. Let us explore the Ayurvedic understanding of the gastrointestinal tract and its interactions with the doshas:

Vata and the Gastrointestinal Tract: Vata dosha is responsible for movement and governs the functions related to the nervous system, muscular movements, and elimination. In the gastrointestinal tract, Vata controls the peristaltic movements that propel food through the digestive system. It also governs the absorption and assimilation of nutrients. When Vata is balanced, the digestive process is smooth, and bowel movements are regular. However, an imbalance in Vata can lead to gas, bloating, and irregular bowel movements, such as constipation or diarrhea.

Pitta and the Gastrointestinal Tract: Pitta dosha represents the fire element and is responsible for transformation and metabolism. In the gastrointestinal tract, Pitta governs the production of digestive enzymes, stomach acid, and bile. These substances aid in the breakdown of food and the absorption of nutrients. Balanced Pitta ensures optimal digestion and assimilation. However, an excess of Pitta can lead to hyperacidity, heartburn, and inflammatory conditions in the digestive tract.

Kapha and the Gastrointestinal Tract: Kapha dosha represents the earth and water elements and is responsible for stability, lubrication, and structural integrity. In the gastrointestinal tract, Kapha provides mucous lining, protecting the digestive system from excess acidity and irritation. It also regulates the moisture content in the digestive system. Balanced Kapha ensures smooth functioning of the gastrointestinal tract and prevents dryness or irritation. However, an imbalance in Kapha can lead to sluggish digestion, heaviness, and mucus-related issues like congestion [2].

2.4 Interactions of Doshas in digestive health

Vata-Pitta Imbalance: Excessive Vata and Pitta imbalances can lead to hyperacidity, indigestion, and inflammation in the gastrointestinal tract. This combination may cause symptoms like burning sensations, gas, and loose stools.

Vata-Kapha Imbalance: A combination of excessive Vata and Kapha can lead to irregular bowel movements, heaviness, and a feeling of incomplete digestion. This imbalance may cause bloating, constipation, and overall digestive discomfort.

Pitta-Kapha Imbalance: When Pitta and Kapha are imbalanced, there can be a tendency for excess mucus production, leading to conditions like gastritis, acidity, and dampness in the digestive tract.

2.5 Ayurvedic approach to maintaining digestive health

Ayurveda emphasizes maintaining a balance among the doshas to ensure optimal digestive health. The following guidelines are often recommended to support digestive wellness:

Eat According to Dosha: Follow a diet that supports your doshic constitution and addresses any imbalances. For example, Vata individuals may benefit from warm, grounding foods, while Pitta individuals may need cooling and soothing foods.

Mindful Eating: Eat in a calm and relaxed environment, savoring each bite mindfully to enhance digestion.

Favor Digestive Spices: Incorporate spices like ginger, cumin, coriander, and fennel, which aid in digestion and balance the doshas.

Maintain a Routine: Follow a regular daily routine, including consistent meal timings, to support the body's natural rhythms and Agni.

Avoid Overeating: Overeating can overload the digestive system and lead to imbalances in the doshas.

Manage Stress: Practice stress-reducing techniques like meditation, yoga, and deep breathing to balance the doshas and support digestion.

Herbal Support: Ayurvedic herbs like Triphala, licorice, and aloe vera are used to support balanced digestion and address specific digestive issues.

By understanding the interactions between the doshas and the gastrointestinal tract, individuals can make informed lifestyle and dietary choices to maintain digestive health and overall well-being according to Ayurvedic principles.

3. Causes and types of constipation in Ayurveda

The various factors that can lead to constipation according to Ayurveda. These may include dietary habits, lifestyle choices, physical inactivity, and psychological factors.

Vata imbalance can significantly disrupt the normal functioning of the colon and lead to constipation in Ayurveda. Vata dosha, being responsible for movement and mobility, plays a crucial role in regulating peristaltic movements, which propel stool through the colon for elimination. When Vata becomes imbalanced, it can lead to irregular and weakened peristaltic movements, causing the stool to become dry and hard, leading to constipation.

3.1 Here's how Vata imbalance can lead to constipation

Dryness: Vata imbalance tends to cause dryness in the body, including the colon. This dryness can lead to inadequate lubrication of the colon, making it difficult for the stool to move smoothly through the intestines.

Irregular Peristaltic Movements: Vata governs the rhythmic contractions of the intestines known as peristalsis. An imbalance in Vata can disrupt these movements, resulting in irregular and sluggish bowel movements.

Nervous System Involvement: Vata is associated with the nervous system. When Vata is imbalanced, it can lead to stress, anxiety, and nervousness, which can further impact the functioning of the gastrointestinal system.

3.2 Different types of constipation based on Dosha imbalance

Vata Predominant Constipation: Dry and hard stools that are difficult to pass Irregular and sluggish bowel movements Abdominal bloating and discomfort Feelings of incomplete evacuation after bowel movements Pitta Predominant Constipation: Infrequent and hard stools with a tendency towards acidity Burning sensation in the abdomen or rectum Increased heat and inflammation in the gastrointestinal tract. A feeling of irritability or frustration related to bowel movements Kapha Predominant Constipation: Heavy and sticky stools that are difficult to eliminate A sense of fullness and heaviness in the abdomen Sluggish and slow bowel movements Excess mucus in the stool or colon Differentiating the types of constipation based on the predominant dosha allows for a more individualized approach to treatment. Treatment strategies for constipation may include:

Vata Predominant Constipation: Focus on lubricating the colon with moistening foods and adequate hydration. Warming spices and gentle exercise can also help stimulate peristalsis.

Pitta Predominant Constipation: Emphasize cooling and soothing foods to reduce inflammation in the gastrointestinal tract. Hydration is essential, and avoiding spicy and acidic foods can be beneficial.

Kapha Predominant Constipation: Focus on foods that promote warmth and lightness to counteract the heavy and sticky qualities of Kapha. Gentle exercises and stimulating spices can aid in promoting regular bowel movements.

Overall, understanding the specific dosha imbalances that contribute to constipation can guide the appropriate lifestyle, dietary, and herbal interventions to address the root cause of the issue and restore balance to the digestive system. It is essential to consult with an experienced Ayurvedic practitioner to receive personalized recommendations for managing constipation based on individual constitution and imbalances.

4. Symptoms and diagnosis of constipation in Ayurveda

In Ayurveda, constipation is viewed as a disturbance in the digestive system that results in the improper elimination of waste products from the body. Observing and understanding bowel movements and stool characteristics are essential in Ayurveda to assess an individual's digestive health and identify imbalances. Several symptoms and indicators can suggest constipation from an Ayurvedic perspective. Here are some common symptoms to look out for:

4.1 Infrequent bowel movements

One of the primary signs of constipation is having infrequent bowel movements. In Ayurveda, regular elimination is considered crucial for maintaining overall health, and a healthy individual should ideally have one or two bowel movements per day [3].

Dry and Hard Stools: Constipation often leads to dry and hard stools. Stools may be difficult to pass, and individuals may experience a sense of incomplete evacuation after a bowel movement.

Straining During Bowel Movements: Difficulty in passing stools can result in straining during bowel movements. This can lead to abdominal discomfort and even rectal bleeding in severe cases.

Abdominal Discomfort: Constipation can cause abdominal discomfort, bloating, and a feeling of heaviness in the stomach area. This discomfort may persist even after bowel movements.

Foul-Smelling Stools: Stools that are not adequately eliminated can lead to a buildup of toxins (Ama) in the digestive tract, resulting in foul-smelling stools.

Coated Tongue: A coated tongue can be an indicator of digestive imbalance, including constipation. The presence of a thick white or yellowish coating on the tongue may suggest poor digestion.

Bad Breath: Poor digestion and constipation can contribute to bad breath or an unpleasant taste in the mouth.

Decreased Appetite: Constipation can cause a decrease in appetite, as the digestive fire (Agni) may become weak or imbalanced.

Fatigue and Lethargy: Chronic constipation can lead to the accumulation of toxins in the body, which may cause fatigue and lethargy.

Irritability and Restlessness: Digestive issues, including constipation, can influence mental well-being, leading to irritability and restlessness.

Emphasizing the observation of bowel movements and stool characteristics is essential in Ayurveda to gain insights into an individual's digestive health. Ayurvedic practitioners often inquire about these factors during consultations to assess the balance of doshas and identify any underlying imbalances. Proper digestion and regular elimination are considered vital for overall health and well-being in Ayurveda.

4.2 To maintain optimal digestive health and prevent constipation, individuals are advised to

Follow a balanced and appropriate diet based on their doshic constitution. Stay well-hydrated throughout the day. Incorporate fiber-rich foods to promote regular bowel movements. Engage in regular physical activity to support digestion. Practice mindfulness during meals and avoid overeating. Manage stress through relaxation techniques, as stress can impact digestion. By paying attention to bowel movements, stool characteristics, and related symptoms, individuals can proactively address constipation and maintain a healthy digestive system according to Ayurvedic principles. If constipation persists or is severe, it is essential to seek guidance from a qualified Ayurvedic practitioner for a personalized treatment plan.

5. Ayurvedic lifestyle practices for constipation prevention

5.1 Practical and holistic lifestyle practices to prevent constipation

Regular Meal Timings: Stick to regular meal timings as per your daily routine. Aim for three main meals (breakfast, lunch, and dinner) and avoid prolonged gaps between meals. This helps maintain a consistent digestive rhythm and prevents irregular bowel movements.

Balanced and Fiber-Rich Diet: Consume a balanced diet that includes a variety of fruits, vegetables, whole grains, legumes, nuts, and seeds. These fiber-rich foods help add bulk to the stool and promote regular bowel movements.

Hydration: Stay well-hydrated throughout the day by drinking an adequate amount of water. Proper hydration helps soften the stool and eases its passage through the colon.

Warm Water in the Morning: Drink a glass of warm water upon waking to stimulate bowel movements and encourage the elimination of waste accumulated overnight.

Herbal Teas: Herbal teas, such as ginger tea or Triphala tea, can aid digestion and promote bowel regularity. Sip on these teas between meals for added benefits.

Avoid Excessive Caffeine and Alcohol: Limit the consumption of caffeine and alcohol, as they can dehydrate the body and potentially contribute to constipation.

Mindful Eating: Practice mindful eating by sitting down to eat in a calm and relaxed environment. Chew your food thoroughly to aid digestion and allow the body to properly assimilate nutrients.

Avoid Overeating and Heavy Meals: Overeating and consuming heavy meals can overwhelm the digestive system and lead to sluggish digestion. Eat until you feel satisfied, not overly full.

Dietary Spices: Incorporate digestion-enhancing spices like ginger, cumin, coriander, and fennel into your meals. These spices can support healthy digestion and help prevent constipation.

Regular Physical Activity: Engage in regular physical activity to promote bowel movements and overall digestive health. Activities like walking, yoga, and gentle exercises can be beneficial.

Daily Routines (Dinacharya): Establish a daily routine that includes consistent meal timings, wake-up times, and bedtime. Following a routine helps the body maintain its natural rhythms, including digestion.

5.2 The significance of daily routines (Dinacharya)

In Ayurveda, daily routines, known as Dinacharya, hold great significance for overall health and well-being. Dinacharya involves aligning your daily activities with the natural rhythms of the day to support the optimal functioning of the body and mind. Here's why daily routines are essential for preventing constipation and maintaining digestive health:

Regulates Digestive Fire (Agni): Following a consistent daily routine helps regulate Agni, the digestive fire. Eating meals at regular intervals and avoiding erratic eating patterns support healthy digestion.

Balances Doshas: Daily routines help balance the doshas, ensuring that Vata, Pitta, and Kapha remain in harmony. Imbalanced doshas can disrupt digestion and lead to constipation.

Syncs with Circadian Rhythms: Aligning your daily routine with the natural cycles of the day, such as waking up and sleeping with the sun, helps synchronize your body's internal clock. This contributes to better digestion and overall well-being.

Reduces Stress: Following a structured daily routine can reduce stress and anxiety, which are known to affect digestive health. Stress can disrupt digestion and contribute to constipation.

Supports Restful Sleep: A consistent daily routine, including a regular bedtime, promotes restful and rejuvenating sleep. Quality sleep is crucial for the body to repair and restore, including proper digestion.

Enhances Mindful Eating: Establishing regular meal times allows you to eat mindfully and pay attention to your body's hunger and satiety cues. This fosters better digestion and prevents overeating.

By incorporating practical and holistic lifestyle practices into your daily routine, you can proactively prevent constipation and support optimal digestive health. Remember that individual needs may vary, so it's essential to personalize these practices based on your doshic constitution and specific health requirements. For personalized guidance, consult with an experienced Ayurvedic practitioner.

6. Ayurvedic herbs and remedies for constipation relief

A comprehensive list of Ayurvedic herbs and remedies used to relieve constipation. The effectiveness of natural laxatives like Triphala, castor oil, and psyllium husk. It includes information on how to prepare and use these remedies safely and effectively.

6.1 Comprehensive list of herbs and remedies

Ayurveda offers a comprehensive list of herbs and remedies that have been traditionally used to relieve constipation. These natural laxatives work by gently stimulating the digestive system, promoting bowel movements, and easing the passage of stools. Let us explore some of the most effective Ayurvedic remedies for constipation relief [4]:

Triphala: Triphala is an Ayurvedic formulation composed of three fruits - Amalaki (Indian Gooseberry), Bibhitaki (Beleric), and Haritaki (Chebulic Myrobalan). It is a well-known and widely used remedy for constipation. Triphala acts as a gentle laxative, helping to cleanse the intestines and promote regular bowel movements. It can be taken in powder form or as a decoction prepared by boiling Triphala powder in water. Preparation and Dosage: Mix 1 teaspoon of Triphala powder in a cup of warm water and let it steep overnight. Drink this decoction in the morning on an empty stomach.

Castor Oil (Erand Taila): Castor oil is a potent natural laxative that acts quickly to relieve constipation. It stimulates the intestines and promotes bowel movements. However, it should be used with caution and not as a regular remedy for constipation, as excessive use can lead to dependency. Preparation and Dosage: Mix 1–2 tablespoons of castor oil in a cup of warm milk or water. Drink it on an empty stomach before bedtime. It is advisable to use castor oil occasionally and not for long-term use.

Psyllium Husk (Isabgol): Psyllium husk is a natural source of soluble fiber and is often used as a bulk-forming laxative. When mixed with water, it swells and forms a gel-like substance that softens the stool and promotes regular bowel movements. Preparation and Dosage: Mix 1–2 teaspoons of psyllium husk in a glass of water or juice and drink it immediately. Follow it with another glass of water to ensure proper hydration.

Haritaki (Chebulic Myrobalan): Haritaki is one of the components of Triphala and can be used independently as a mild laxative. It has gentle effects on the digestive system and helps relieve constipation. Preparation and Dosage: Soak 2–3 haritaki fruits in water overnight. Drink the water in the morning on an empty stomach.

Aloe Vera: Aloe vera gel has a soothing effect on the digestive tract and can help soften the stool, making it easier to pass. Aloe vera juice is used occasionally for constipation relief. Preparation and Dosage: Mix 1–2 tablespoons of aloe vera gel in a glass of water or juice and drink it on an empty stomach.

Senna: Senna leaves have potent laxative properties and are commonly used for acute constipation relief. However, they should be used sparingly and under the guidance of an experienced practitioner, as prolonged use may lead to dependency.

Preparation and Dosage: Senna leaves are available in the form of tea or as capsules. Follow the recommended dosage on the packaging or as advised by a healthcare professional [4].

6.2 Safety and precautions

Always consult with a qualified Ayurvedic practitioner or healthcare professional before using any laxative remedies, especially if you are pregnant, nursing, or have underlying health conditions. Natural laxatives should be used occasionally and not as a long-term solution for constipation. Ensure adequate hydration when using fiber-based laxatives like psyllium husk to prevent dehydration. Avoid using harsh laxatives like senna for extended periods, as they may cause dependency and disrupt natural bowel function. Incorporating these Ayurvedic remedies into your routine can provide gentle and effective relief from constipation. However, remember that individual responses to these remedies may vary, so it's crucial to find what works best for your body and doshic constitution. Always seek personalized guidance to ensure safe and effective use of these herbal remedies.

7. Yoga and Pranayama for constipation management

The specific asanas and pranayama techniques can aid in managing constipation. Explain how yoga postures like Pawanmuktasana (Wind-Relieving Pose) and Malasana (Squatting Pose) can stimulate bowel movements and reduce Vata imbalances. The practice of Nadi Shodhana (Alternate Nostril Breathing) is to calm the mind and balance the doshas.

7.1 Specific Yogasana and Pranayama techniques for managing constipation

Yoga, including specific asanas (postures) and pranayama (breathing techniques), can be beneficial in managing constipation by promoting healthy digestion, stimulating the abdominal organs, and relieving digestive discomfort. Here are some specific yoga practices that can aid in managing constipation [5]:

Asanas (Yoga Poses): [6].

Pawanmuktasana (Wind-Relieving Pose): Pawanmuktasana helps in releasing excess gas from the abdomen, relieving bloating, and promoting bowel movements. It also stretches the lower back and hips. How to do it:

Lie on your back with legs straight. Exhale and bring your right knee towards your chest, clasping your hands around it. Inhale, lift your head and chest towards your knee. Exhale and release the pose. Repeat with the left knee. Malasana (Garland Pose): Malasana helps in stretching the lower back and opening the hips, which can aid in relieving constipation by encouraging smooth bowel movements.

How to do it: Squat down with your feet wider than hip-width apart. Bring your palms together in a prayer position and gently push your elbows against your inner thighs. Stay in this pose for a few breaths. Uttanasana (Standing Forward Bend): Uttanasana helps in stretching the hamstrings, lower back, and abdominal muscles, improving blood flow to the pelvic region and stimulating digestion.

How to do it: Stand with your feet hip-width apart. Inhale, lengthen your spine, and as you exhale, bend forward from your hips, reaching your hands towards the floor or your shins. Hold the pose for a few breaths. Pranayama (Breathing Techniques):

Kapalabhati Pranayama (Skull-Shining Breath): Kapalabhati is a cleansing and energizing breath that helps in stimulating the abdominal organs and improving digestion.

How to do it: Sit in a comfortable cross-legged position. Take a deep breath in and then forcefully exhale by contracting your abdominal muscles. Allow the inhalation to happen passively. Repeat this rapid exhalation-inhalation cycle for 30–60 seconds, and then take a deep breath to relax. Nadi Shodhana Pranayama (Alternate Nostril Breathing): Nadi Shodhana helps in balancing the energy flow in the body and calming the mind. It also aids in reducing stress, which can impact digestion.

How to do it: Sit comfortably with a straight spine. Use your right thumb to close your right nostril and inhale deeply through your left nostril. Use your right ring finger to close your left nostril and exhale through your right nostril. Inhale through your right nostril, close it with your right thumb, and exhale through your left nostril. This completes one round. Continue for a few minutes. Remember to practice yoga mindfully and within your body's limitations. If you have any pre-existing health conditions or concerns, consult with a yoga instructor or healthcare professional before starting a new yoga practice. Yoga can be a valuable complementary approach to managing constipation when combined with a balanced diet, adequate hydration, and other lifestyle adjustments.

8. Ayurvedic dietary guidelines for constipation relief

This chapter provides in-depth guidance on dietary modifications for constipation relief. The role of fiber-rich foods, spices, and herbal teas in promoting healthy digestion.

8.1 Dietary guidelines

Dietary modifications play a crucial role in managing constipation and promoting healthy digestion in Ayurveda. The right combination of foods can help regulate bowel movements, improve gut health, and prevent digestive discomfort [7]. Here's in-depth guidance on dietary modifications for constipation relief:

Include Fiber-Rich Foods: Fiber adds bulk to the stool and helps in its smooth passage through the digestive tract. Include the following fiber-rich foods in your diet: Whole Grains: Brown rice, quinoa, oats, barley, and whole wheat are excellent sources of dietary fiber. Fruits: Apples, pears, berries, prunes, and figs are high in soluble and insoluble fiber. Vegetables: Leafy greens, broccoli, carrots, beets, and sweet potatoes are fiber-rich options. Legumes: Lentils, chickpeas, black beans, and kidney beans are great sources of fiber. Stay Hydrated: Adequate hydration is essential for softening the stool and supporting regular bowel movements. Drink plenty of water throughout the day. Herbal teas, coconut water, and fresh fruit juices are also hydrating options.

Consume Healthy Fats: Healthy fats, such as ghee (clarified butter), coconut oil, and olive oil, help lubricate the intestines and promote bowel regularity.

Emphasize Digestion-Enhancing Spices: Incorporate digestion-enhancing spices into your meals, as they aid in promoting healthy digestion and preventing constipation. Some beneficial spices include:

Ginger: It improves digestion, reduces gas, and soothes the digestive tract. Cumin: It aids in digestion, relieves bloating, and promotes bowel movements. Coriander: It has carminative properties that alleviate gas and indigestion. Fennel: It relieves digestive discomfort, bloating, and constipation. Herbal Teas for Digestive Health: Herbal teas can have soothing and digestive benefits. Consider the following herbal teas for promoting healthy digestion: Peppermint Tea: It relaxes the gastrointestinal muscles and eases digestive discomfort. Ginger Tea: It aids in digestion, reduces inflammation, and improves gut health. Licorice Tea: It soothes the digestive tract and helps in relieving constipation. Chew Your Food Thoroughly: Chewing food thoroughly allows for better digestion and nutrient absorption. It also helps in breaking down food particles, making it easier for the digestive system to process.

Avoid Processed and Junk Foods: Processed foods, fried foods, and high-fat items can slow down digestion and contribute to constipation. Limit their consumption and opt for whole, unprocessed foods.

Regular Meal Timings: Eating meals at consistent times each day helps regulate the body's natural digestive rhythm, promoting regular bowel movements.

Mindful Eating: Eat in a calm and relaxed environment, avoiding distractions. Pay attention to your food, chew mindfully, and savor each bite to aid digestion.

Triphala for Constipation: Triphala, a combination of three fruits, is an excellent Ayurvedic herbal remedy for constipation relief. It can be taken as a powder or in capsule form. Triphala helps regulate bowel movements and promotes healthy digestion.

Remember that individual responses to dietary modifications may vary based on dosha imbalances and overall health. It's essential to consult with an experienced Ayurvedic practitioner or healthcare professional to receive personalized dietary recommendations for constipation relief and overall digestive health. Combining these dietary modifications with other lifestyle practices, including regular exercise and stress management, can enhance the effectiveness of constipation management strategies.

9. Ayurvedic detoxification for colon health

The concept of Panchakarma, a comprehensive Ayurvedic detoxification procedure, and its role in maintaining colon health. The specific Panchakarma therapies that target constipation and cleanse the gastrointestinal tract. It emphasizes the need for qualified Ayurvedic practitioners to administer Panchakarma treatments.

9.1 Ayurvedic detoxification procedure

Panchakarma is a comprehensive Ayurvedic detoxification and rejuvenation procedure aimed at purifying the body, mind, and soul. The term "Panchakarma" is derived from the Sanskrit words "Pancha" (five) and "Karma" (actions), referring to the five therapeutic actions that constitute the treatment. It is an intricate and highly personalized process that involves several therapeutic procedures to remove accumulated toxins (Ama) and restore balance to the doshas.

9.2 The role of Panchakarma in maintaining colon health

In Ayurveda, the colon (large intestine) plays a vital role in eliminating waste materials from the body. An accumulation of toxins and imbalances in the gastrointestinal tract can lead to constipation, digestive issues, and other health problems.

Panchakarma focuses on cleansing and rejuvenating the digestive system, including the colon, to promote optimal digestive health. By removing Ama and restoring balance to the doshas, Panchakarma supports the natural healing and revitalization of the colon.

9.3 Specific Panchakarma therapies for constipation and gastrointestinal cleansing

Virechana (Purgation Therapy): Virechana is a therapeutic purgation process that involves the administration of a specific herbal purgative to cleanse the intestines and eliminate excess Pitta and toxins. It is particularly beneficial for Pitta imbalances and conditions like constipation, acidity, and inflammation in the gastrointestinal tract. Virechana helps in clearing accumulated Ama and promoting healthy bowel movements.

Basti (Enema Therapy): Basti is an essential Panchakarma therapy that involves the introduction of herbal decoctions and oils into the rectum to cleanse the colon and balance the Vata dosha. This therapy is highly effective for Vata-related constipation, as it lubricates the intestines, softens the stool, and facilitates easy elimination. Basti is also beneficial for promoting overall digestive health and relieving digestive disorders.

Abhyanga (Ayurvedic Oil Massage): Abhyanga is a full-body massage using warm herbal oils, which helps in promoting blood circulation, relaxing the muscles, and calming the nervous system. This preparation is essential before undergoing the other Panchakarma therapies, as it helps in mobilizing toxins from the tissues and directing them towards the gastrointestinal tract for elimination.

Nasya (Nasal Administration of Medicines): Nasya involves the application of herbal oils or medicated powders into the nostrils. It helps in clearing the nasal passages, sinuses, and head region, balancing the Kapha dosha, and facilitating proper drainage of fluids, which indirectly affects gastrointestinal health.

Herbal Steam Therapy: Swedana or herbal steam therapy is used to open up the channels, release toxins, and facilitate the elimination of impurities through sweat. Steam therapy can be employed before or after other Panchakarma procedures to enhance their effectiveness.

It's important to note that Panchakarma is a specialized and intensive Ayurvedic therapy that requires proper assessment and guidance from a qualified Ayurvedic practitioner. The specific therapies chosen for an individual will depend on their doshic constitution, the nature of the imbalance, and other health considerations. Panchakarma should only be undertaken under the supervision of a trained practitioner to ensure its safe and effective implementation. When conducted properly, Panchakarma can be a powerful tool for maintaining colon health, promoting digestive well-being, and supporting overall rejuvenation of the body and mind.

10. Ayurvedic psychology and stress management

The connection between emotional imbalances, stress, and constipation in Ayurveda. It also provides insights into how stress affects the doshas and disrupts normal bowel movements. Offer Ayurvedic approaches to managing stress through meditation, mindfulness, and herbal supplements.

10.1 Emotional imbalances, stress, and constipation in Ayurveda

In Ayurveda, the mind and body are intimately interconnected, and emotional imbalances, particularly stress, can significantly impact the doshas and disrupt normal bowel movements. Ayurvedic texts emphasize the role of mental well-being in maintaining overall health, including digestive health. The connection between emotional imbalances, stress, and constipation can be understood through the lens of dosha imbalances [8, 9]:

Vata Dosha Imbalance: Stress and emotional upheavals are known to disturb Vata dosha, which governs movement, including the movement of the intestines and the elimination of waste. When Vata is imbalanced due to stress, it can lead to irregular and sluggish bowel movements, resulting in constipation. Additionally, stress can cause the nervous system to be in a constant state of fight-or-flight response, leading to increased tension and constriction in the gastrointestinal tract, further contributing to constipation.

Agni (Digestive Fire) Imbalance: Stress and emotional disturbances can weaken Agni, the digestive fire. When Agni is weakened, it leads to improper digestion and inadequate breakdown of food, resulting in the formation of Ama (toxins). Accumulated Ama can disrupt the normal functioning of the colon and lead to constipation.

Kapha Dosha Imbalance: Although Kapha dosha is not directly associated with stress, prolonged stress can lead to imbalances in all three doshas, including Kapha. Kapha imbalances can cause heaviness, sluggishness, and reduced motility in the gastrointestinal tract, contributing to constipation.

Impact on Gut-Brain Axis: The gut-brain axis is a complex communication network between the gut and the brain. Stress can negatively affect this axis, leading to changes in gut motility, secretion, and sensitivity. This disruption can lead to alterations in bowel movements and contribute to constipation.

Nervous System Imbalance: Stress activates the sympathetic nervous system (fight-or-flight response) and inhibits the parasympathetic nervous system (rest-and-digest response). This imbalance can slow down digestive functions, including peristalsis (contractions that move stool through the intestines), leading to constipation.

Psychological Factors: Emotional imbalances, such as anxiety, fear, and worry, can create mental tension, which affects the autonomic nervous system and further exacerbates constipation. Negative emotions can lead to poor eating habits, irregular meal timings, and inadequate hydration, all of which can contribute to digestive issues.

10.2 Addressing stress and emotional imbalances for constipation relief

To manage constipation effectively in Ayurveda, it is essential to address stress and emotional imbalances. Here are some Ayurvedic strategies to help:

Practice Stress-Relief Techniques: Meditation, yoga, pranayama, and mindfulness practices can help reduce stress and promote relaxation, supporting a balanced nervous system and healthy digestion.

Adopt a Mindful Approach to Eating: Mindful eating, in a calm and relaxed environment, can aid in proper digestion and prevent overeating.

Herbal Support: Ayurvedic herbs like Ashwagandha, Brahmi, and Jatamansi can help reduce stress and balance the doshas.

Regular Daily Routine: Maintain a consistent daily routine, including regular meal timings, exercise, and sleep patterns, to support the body's natural rhythms.

DOI: http://dx.doi.org/10.5772/intechopen.1003646

Seek Emotional Support: Talk to a counselor, therapist, or support group to address emotional imbalances and stress.

Ayurvedic Doctors: Consider Ayurvedic Doctors such as Abhyanga (oil massage), Shirodhara (oil pouring on the forehead), and Nasya (nasal administration of medicated oils) to calm the mind and balance the doshas.

By addressing emotional imbalances and stress, individuals can support their digestive health and reduce the occurrence of constipation. An integrative approach that combines Ayurvedic principles, stress management, and lifestyle modifications can provide effective relief and promote overall well-being. As always, it is essential to consult with an experienced Ayurvedic practitioner for personalized guidance and treatment.

11. Conclusion

In conclusion, constipation, known as Malavastambha in Ayurveda, is a prevalent digestive issue that affects people of all age groups and significantly impacts their quality of life. It disrupts the normal functioning of the digestive system, leading to various negative effects.

Ayurveda, the ancient holistic healing system, views constipation as a manifestation of an imbalance in the Vata dosha, responsible for governing movement and elimination in the body. This unique perspective provides valuable insights into the root causes, symptoms, and effective treatment strategies for constipation.

By understanding constipation from the Ayurvedic standpoint, individuals gain access to a holistic and natural approach to alleviate this ailment. Ayurveda emphasizes restoring balance not only in the physical body but also in the mind and spirit, recognizing the interconnectedness of these elements for overall wellness.

Ayurvedic management of constipation involves dietary adjustments, lifestyle modifications, herbal remedies, therapeutic practices, and even specialized treatments like Basti (enema). These approaches not only provide relief from constipation but also promote the well-being of the entire individual.

In adopting Ayurvedic principles for constipation management, individuals can move towards a state of equilibrium in their digestive system and experience improved health and vitality. This ancient system of healing encourages us to look beyond mere symptom relief and address the underlying imbalances that lead to constipation, ultimately supporting a more harmonious and fulfilling life.

Author details

Shweta Parwe[1,2]* and Milind Nisargandha[3]

1 Department of Panchakarma, Mahatma Gandhi Ayurved College, Hospital and Research Centre, Wardha, India

2 Datta Meghe Institute of Higher Education and Research (D.M.I.H.E.R.) (D.U.), Wardha, Maharashtra, India

3 Saveetha Medical College and Hospital, Saveetha Institute of Medical and Technical Sciences, Saveetha University, Chennai, India

*Address all correspondence to: drshwetaparve@gmail.com

References

[1] Agrawal A, Yadav CR, Meena MS. Physiological aspects of Agni. Ayu. 2010;**31**(3):395

[2] Rizvi SAA, Einstein GP, Tulp OL, Sainvil F, Branly R. Introduction to traditional medicine and their role in prevention and treatment of emerging and Re-emerging diseases. Biomolecules. 2022;**12**(10):1442

[3] Singh SK, Rajoria K. Ayurvedic management of chronic constipation in Hirschsprung disease – A case study. Journal of Ayurveda and Integrative Medicine. 2018;**9**(2):131-135

[4] Hoffmann D. Healthy Digestion A Natural Approach to Relieving Indigestion. Gas, Heartburn, Constipation, Colitis, and More. Hachette, UK: Storey Publishing, LLC; 2017

[5] Kavuri V, Raghuram N, Malamud A, Selvan SR. Irritable bowel syndrome: Yoga as remedial therapy. Evidence-Based Complementary and Alternative Medicine. 2015;**2015**

[6] Saraswati SS, Hiti JK. Asana Pranayama Mudra Bandha. Bihar, India: Yoga Publications Trust; 1996

[7] Rawat S, Singh R, Sahu P, Padhar BK, Mutha R, Meena HML. A conceptual study of Grahani Roga (irritable bowel syndrome) and its management through dietary modification. International Research Journal of Ayurveda & Yoga. 2022;**05**(02):99-104

[8] Khalsa SB, Cohen L, Mccall T, Telles S. Principles and Practice of Yoga in Health Care. London: Jessica Kingsley Publishers; 2016

[9] Kumar N, Bowling M. Ayurvedic medicine in children and adolescents. In: Handbook of Mind/Body Integration in Child and Adolescent Development. Cham: Springer International Publishing; 2023